Fitness Nutrition

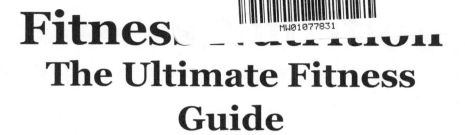

The Ultimate Fitness Guide

Health, Fitness, Nutrition, and Muscle Building

Lose Weight and Build Lean Muscle

5th Edition

By

Nicholas Bjorn

Nicholas Bjorn

author is not engaging in the rendering of legal, financial, medical, or professional advice.

Table of Contents

Introduction

I want to thank you and congratulate you for purchasing the book, "Fitness Nutrition: The Ultimate Fitness Guide: Health, Fitness, Nutrition and Muscle Building – Lose Weight and Build Lean Muscle." This book contains proven steps and strategies on how to lose weight and build lean muscle naturally and safely, all through nutrition.

The foods we eat are just as important as working out and exercising, if not more. This book will introduce you to important information about what types of foods you should be eating to help you achieve your fitness goals. We will look at how different foods affect your body in terms of providing energy and nutrients, as well as which types of foods and food components should be avoided due to the negative impact that they can have on your health. You will also learn all about carbohydrates, fats, and proteins and how to choose the right foods to achieve weight loss and build lean muscle. We will discuss how to determine your caloric requirements both to maintain your weight and to lose weight if that is your goal. Moreover, in this book, you will learn exactly how calories work and the importance of limiting your portions.

Once you have a more in-depth understanding of how the food that you eat will affect your health and fitness levels, as well as how to eat to achieve the best results, we will move to the exercise portion of the book. This book also contains plenty of effective fitness nutrition tips and exercises that will guide you toward achieving your health and fitness goals. You will learn about a variety of different exercises that can help you build lean muscle mass and improve your overall fitness level. We will discuss exercises that target each core muscle area of your body so that you can make sure that your entire body is getting the exercise and strengthening that it needs. Whether you are working out in a gym, outside, or in your own home, this book will provide exercises that you can use in a way that is easy to follow and understand.

After you have the nutritional basics under control and have an idea of some exercises that you can do to improve your fitness level and build lean muscle mass, we will take a look at some recipe ideas. These recipes can be added to your diet to make sure that it is as healthy as possible while following your caloric requirements, whether your goal is to maintain or lose weight.

This book will then take you through a more in-depth discussion of what to avoid, both in terms of exercising and diet. It is important to ensure that you are exercising and eating in a way that will improve your health and well-being while avoiding anything in your diet or your activities that will impede your health goals or cause negative health effects.

One of the last chapters in this book will provide you with some ideas on how to stick to your diet and exercise plan, even while you are on vacation, and still enjoy yourself. We all know how tempting it is to vary from your exercise and nutritional goals while you are on vacation, which can make it difficult to return to your plan when you get back from vacation. The tips and tricks in this book will help you avoid that scenario, such that you stick to your diet and exercise plan while you are away. This enables you to feel as healthy as possible on vacation while preventing yourself from deviating from your health and fitness goals.

Once you have read this book, you will have a much better understanding of your nutritional requirements and how to eat so that you are giving your body its best chance at being as healthy as possible. You will also have learned how to exercise so that you can achieve all of your fitness goals. Make sure to go back through the book from time to time so that you remember all of the important pieces of information and ensure that you are maintaining the best possible diet and exercise plan.

Thanks again for purchasing this book. I hope you enjoy it!

Nicholas Bjorn

FREE E-BOOKS SENT WEEKLY

Join <u>North Star Readers Book Club</u>
And Get Exclusive Access To The Latest Kindle Books in
Fitness, Health, Weight Loss and Much More…

TO GET YOU STARTED HERE IS YOUR FREE E-BOOK:

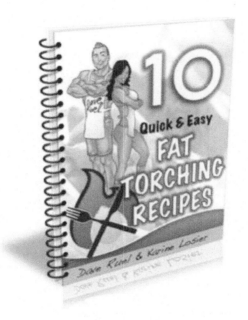

Visit to Sign Up Today!

www.northstarreaders.com/10-fat-torching-recipes

Nicholas Bjorn

Chapter 1: How Calories Work

In this day and age, where life has become just so hectic, there is hardly any time for people to stop and look at their diet. From consuming sugary foods to fat-laden junk, everybody is now only interested in satiating their hunger and going about their daily activities. But then, what really are the long-term consequences of following such a diet?

Well, for starters, people will begin to turn obese and acquire various illnesses, both mental and physical in nature. There are many serious health consequences that arise from being overweight, including heart problems, high blood pressure, stroke, diabetes, cancer, osteoarthritis, and sleep apnea. Coronary heart disease is one of the most significant possible health impacts: as your body mass index (which will be discussed in a later chapter) increases, so does your risk of suffering from coronary heart disease. Coronary heart disease involves plaque building up inside your coronary arteries, which are the arteries that move oxygen-rich blood to your heart. If blood flow to the heart is reduced, this can cause angina (chest pain) or a heart attack. If the plaque buildup reaches a certain level, it can cause heart failure. If an area of plaque ruptures, this can cause a blood clot to form, which in turn can cause a stroke.

The development of Type-II Diabetes is another serious health issue that can arise as a result of being overweight. The insulin produced by your body allows the breakdown of sugar so that it can be stored or burned by your body as necessary. Excess body fat leads to an increased likelihood of insulin resistance, which means that your body is not able to break down the sugar that you eat. This will eventually lead to the development of Type-II Diabetes.

Being overweight can also lead to increased risk of certain types of cancer, including cancer of the pancreas, breast, colon, kidney, thyroid, and gallbladder.

As indicated above, these are just some of the serious physical health issues that can arise from being overweight. There can also be mental health impacts: depression and anxiety, in particular, can develop as a result of being overweight, along with the feeling of helplessness or loss of control associated with increased weight gain.

Add to these physical and mental health issues the ill effects of a sedentary lifestyle and stress, and you have the perfect recipe for disaster. The need of the hour is, therefore, to make appropriate food choices and try and get your health back on the right track. That is the primary goal. Once it is attained, the priority changes. It becomes primary to build lean muscles so that you don't go back to your old habits and become obese again.

You have to follow a strict diet and an exercise program that allows you to control the amount of calorie intake and manage to build lean muscles. All these and more is covered in this book, and I hope you treat it as your one true lean muscle-building guide.

Any effective weight loss diet follows this simple rule: eat less, and burn more calories. So what is a calorie? Understanding this will show you the crucial role that nutrition plays in losing weight and gaining lean muscle.

What Calories Are

The dictionary definition of a "calorie" is this: it is a unit or quantity of heat that is needed to raise the temperature of 1 gram of water by 1 degree Celsius (or 1.8 degrees Fahrenheit) at atmospheric pressure.

The "calories" used in food are actually kilocalories, and 1 kilocalorie is equal to 1,000 calories. This means that if a box of cookies has 140 calories per serving; it actually means 140,000 actual calories. Nutritionists use the word "calories" to describe the energy-producing potential in food, and it is these calories that fuel all of our bodily functions.

The "calories" in exercise also means the same: if a fitness chart states that you will burn 100 calories for each mile that you run, it actually means you burn 100,000 calories or 100 kilocalories. Hence, when the word "calorie" is mentioned in this book, it refers to kilocalories.

Calories have received a somewhat negative reputation in recent decades, thanks to various fad diets and the tendency to discuss calories as unwanted things. In reality, calories are essential to our survival: if we do not eat enough calories on a daily basis, our bodies will not have the energy required to continue to function, and eventually, our bodies would break down. The important factor is knowing how many calories you are eating and how many you are burning and then making sure that you are not eating more than you are burning – this will help you avoid weight gain while maintaining a healthy lifestyle.

Breaking Down Calories In Food

The number of calories in your food shows the amount of energy that you will get from it. All foods are a combination of three building blocks, and these are carbohydrates, protein, and fat, all of which are referred to as macronutrients. The calories in each macronutrient are as follows:

- **Carbohydrates** – 4 calories

- **Protein** – 4 calories

- **Fat** – 9 calories

As fat has more than twice the amount of calories as carbohydrates and protein, it obviously means fat is more difficult to burn off. Therefore, it should be consumed sparingly.

Let's take a look at the nutritional label on a box of cookies, which shows that the serving size is 25 grams, and the amount of calories per serving is 120. If we open up the packet and burn up the cookies directly in an open fire and let it burn off entirely, this will produce 120 kilocalories, which is enough to increase the temperature of 120 kilograms of water to 1 degree Celsius.

A closer look at the nutritional label will show you that there are 5 grams of fat, 16 grams of carbohydrates, and 3 grams of protein, which gives you a total of 24 grams (food companies tend to round off the amount). Therefore, the 120 calories on the nutrition label of the cookies actually contain 45 calories from fat (5 grams multiplied by 9 calories), 64 calories from carbohydrates, and 12 calories from protein.

For the body to burn these 120 calories, it has to break down the carbohydrates into sugars, such as glucose, the proteins into amino acids, and the fats into fatty acids and glycerol. After this, these organic compounds are transferred via the bloodstream to the different cells in the body for immediate use, and the excess would be stored for future use in the form of body fat.

Sugars, proteins, and fats are each broken down by the body into different compounds, which are then used by the body for different functions. Carbohydrates are broken down by your body into glucose, which is then absorbed through the walls of the small intestine. The glucose is processed by the liver. It then enters the body's circulatory system, increasing the body's blood glucose levels. This provides the body with an excellent (and quickly accessed) source of energy. If there is excess glucose, the liver will store it to be used between mealtimes if the blood glucose levels fall below a certain level. Any glucose in excess of what the liver can store will be turned into fat to be stored for the long term.

Proteins, on the other hand, are broken down into amino acids, which are used by the body to build new proteins. Each of these proteins has a specific function, such as enabling chemical reactions or allowing cells to communicate. If the body is low in glucose and fatty acids, then the body can get energy from protein, but this is not ideal.

Finally, fat is broken down by the body into fatty acids, which are burned as energy. Fatty acids make a fantastic energy source for the body, although it is important to note that not all cells can use fatty acids for energy; brain cells, for example, do require glucose, so be careful when thinking about limiting your carbohydrate intake. If more fatty acids are broken down than the body needs for energy at that moment, then the fatty acids are packaged together in bundles called triglycerides and then stored in fat cells for use at a later date.

Proteins, fats, and sugars each play an important role in the body, and it is essential to ensure that you are taking in enough of each so that your body has the energy and other resources that it needs to carry out all of its functions.

Our Daily Caloric Needs

When nutritional labels show the percentages of the daily values that the body needs, they typically refer to someone who follows a 2,000-calorie diet. It is difficult to identify exactly how many calories our cells require to function properly, as each person's daily physical activities vary, along with his or her height, weight, age, and gender. This is why it is more helpful to look at the amount of calories listed on the nutritional label rather than the percentage of the daily diet.

To know approximately how many calories you need to consume per day so that you can achieve your weight loss goals, there are three important factors that you need to be aware of:

1. **Basal Metabolic Rate or BMR**

2. **Physical Activity**

3. **Thermic Effect Of Food**

These three factors need to be calculated, and by adding up the calculations from these, the result would be the total amount of calories that your body requires each day. There are many calorie counters available online, all of which give different results based on the formulas they used. Adding the above three factors is the most accurate way of determining how many calories your body requires each day.

Here's a starting point for the number of calories you should be eating if you live a sedentary lifestyle.

For men (to maintain weight):

Ages 19–30 should eat anywhere from 2,400 to 2,600.

Ages 31–50 should eat anywhere from 2,200 to 2,400.

Ages 51 and up should eat anywhere from 2,000 to 2,200.

For women (to maintain weight):

Recommended 1,600 to 2,000.

Keep in mind that these are simply starting points. They will only be able to get you so far, so you will need to get an individualized number of calories to eat every day. It changes if you want to lose, gain, or maintain your weight depending on your lifestyle, which is why it is important to calculate it yourself.

Basal Metabolic Rate (BMR)

A person's BMR refers to the amount of energy required for his or her body to function while at rest; that is to say, for the lungs to continue breathing, the heart to keep pumping, the kidneys to keep functioning, and the body temperature to remain stable. These functions take up approximately 60 to 70 percent of the calories that are burned during the day. On average, the BMR of men is higher than that of women.

To estimate your BMR, what you can do is to follow the Harris–Benedict formula:

For adult men: 66 + (6.3 x body weight in pounds) + (12.9 x height in inches) – (6.8 x age in years)

For adult women: 655 + (4.3 x weight in pounds) + (4.7 x height in inches) – (4.7 x age in years)

It might look unusual for men to have 66 and for women to have 655 as the first digits in the formula, but this, in fact, is accurate.

Age is an important factor in the formula because BMR tends to decline by 1% to 2% per decade after you turn 20, largely due to continued loss of fat-free mass in the body. This is, of course, a generalization, and it can differ among individuals depending on exercise, diet, and a person's percentage of body fat.

Increases in muscle mass will also increase your BMR, so if you have calculated your BMR previously and then started an exercise regime that has increased your muscle mass, you should recalculate to make sure that you have a current and correct idea of your BMR.

Another equation that can be used to calculate your BMR, which has been found to be approximately 5% more accurate than the Harris–Benedict formula, is the Mifflin St. Jeor Equation:

For adult men: (10 x weight in kg) + (6.25 x height in cm) – (5 x age in years) + 5

For adult women: (10 x weight in kg) + (6.25 x height in cm) – (5 x age in years) – 161.

If you know your body fat percentage, you can also use the Katch–McArdle formula:

For adult men and women: (21.6 x fat free mass) + 370, where "fat free mass" = weight − (body fat percentage x weight)

The important thing to remember is that each individual is different, and each of these formulas will work better for some and not as well for others. If you have concerns about whether you are using the right formula, or if you are properly calculating your BMR, then you should seek your doctor's assistance.

Physical Activity

After BMR, this is the second main factor that burns considerable amounts of calories. This includes all that you do with your body, such as walking to work, swimming at the pool, and talking to your friend. The amount of calories that are burned off from physical activity actually depends on your body weight. The more weight you have, the more calories you actually burn off as you engage in a particular physical activity. However, if you keep eating as many calories (if not more) as you burn off, you will continue to maintain your current weight (if not increase it).

A great tool to use to calculate how many calories each activity burns is at bitelog.com/exercise-search.htm, but there are many online resources that can you help you to figure out how many calories you are burning.

While many people automatically think of activities like running or going to the gym as the best options for burning calories, there are many other activities that you can choose that will do a great job of burning calories. If you are one of those people who prefer to disguise their exercise in a fun activity, some of these options will work well for you.

Hiking and rock climbing are two excellent examples of fun, outdoor activities that will also help you to burn a large amount of calories. Depending on the difficulty of the trail and how quickly you are walking, you can burn around 400 calories per hour while hiking, whereas rock climbing can burn from 500 to 700 calories per hour. The difference in calories burned for rock climbing comes from how much you weigh because you are using your own body as the weight in this exercise. On days when the weather is not great, indoor rock climbing is always a great alternative.

If you have some household chores that need to get done and think you don't have time to exercise, think again: those chores are exercise! Vacuuming, laundry, sweeping, and mopping will all burn calories, and using those online resources mentioned earlier can help you figure out just how many calories each chore will burn. If you need to wash your car, that will burn about 200 calories per hour, and mowing the lawn (using a push mower, not a riding mower!) will burn around 300 calories per hour. Checking items off the "to-do list" and burning calories both make this option a great combination.

Playing sports is perhaps an obvious way to burn calories, but it still should be mentioned because it's a great way to have fun with your friends and still get your exercise in. Football can burn around 500 calories per hour, assuming that you and your friends are somewhat serious about the game, while soccer can burn 600 calories or even more per hour. Even badminton, which is a much lower impact sport, can burn between 250 and 400 calories depending on how much you weigh.

Yoga is an excellent option because aside from burning calories (around 300 per hour), it also provides a variety of other health benefits: core strength, balance, and flexibility. Plus, it can be very soothing if you are feeling stressed out or wanting to give your body a rest from more strenuous activities.

Thermic Effect Of Food

This is the last factor that burns the calories that you consume, and it is the amount of energy that the body utilizes in order to digest the food that you have consumed. After all, it does take energy to digest the foods and then break them down to the basic organic compounds that the cells need in order to function properly.

To determine the amount of calories that your body utilizes for this, what you do is multiply the total number of calories consumed within a day by 10 percent.

Exercise And Calories

When you eat a total of 3,500 more calories in a week, you will gain one pound of fat. Therefore the only way to get rid of this is by burning 3,500 calories more than what you consume in a week by reducing your portions, increasing your physical activity, or both. Burning 3,500 calories in a week will result in a 1 lb loss in body weight. It is the only way to naturally change a pound of fat into energy.

The beauty of exercise lies in its ability to boost your metabolic rate even though you have stopped doing the physical activity. Metabolism takes time to revert to its regular rate, which is why the body continues to burn calories for the next 120 minutes after exercising.

Nutrition And Calories

If weight loss was the only concern, then you would only have to count the calories. It wouldn't matter whether it is a carbohydrate, protein, or fat calorie. But as much as you need to focus on burning more calories than what you consume, you also need to focus on the nutritional value of the foods. Carbohydrates and proteins are better calorie sources than fats, even though the body does need fat to help absorb fat-soluble vitamins, such as vitamin A. Ideally, you should not eat foods that contain more than 25 to 30 percent of fat calories.

Chapter 2: Choose Carbohydrates Wisely

Carbohydrates are the first building blocks of food, and understanding how they work will help you choose your sources of nutrients effectively to promote weight loss and build lean muscle.

How Carbohydrates Are Converted Into Energy

After eating carbohydrates, your body breaks them down into sugars, which cause your blood glucose level to increase. As this happens, the pancreas releases insulin, which is an anabolic hormone responsible for transporting nutrients into the muscle cells and helping muscles recover. The second function of insulin is to eliminate surplus glucose from the blood and shuttle it into liver glycogen or muscle glycogen stores. However, if both the liver and muscle glycogen stores have been maximized, the surplus blood glucose will then be stored as fat.

When you exercise, muscle glycogen stores are utilized, and the corresponding insulin released when eating high-carbohydrate foods will cause the surplus blood glucose, along with the rest of the nutrients, to be shuttled into the muscle cells. This boosts muscle protein synthesis and muscle recovery, which in turn builds lean muscle.

As you know, that is your ultimate goal. You are taking up these exercises because you wish to have lean muscles at the end of it all. Once you have your goals set, it becomes increasingly easy for you to follow and pursue them. Thus, it is important to do as many "right" things as possible in order to attain your goal faster. So be wise in choosing what you put inside your body in terms of carbs. This is further explained in detail under the next heading.

The Importance Of Quantity And Quality

The level of increase in your blood sugar from the consumption of carbohydrates greatly depends on the amount that you consume, as well as how quickly the carbohydrates are digested. The amount of fiber in the carbohydrates, as well as fat and protein content, is also a major factor.

In order to lose weight and boost muscle recovery from carbohydrate consumption, it is best to choose food sources that are unrefined and rich in fiber. This will ensure that the carbohydrate will be digested more slowly, leading to steadier blood sugar increase and insulin response. Refined starches and sugars from which fiber is removed become easily digested and trigger an immediate blood sugar spike, followed by a crash once the insulin plays its role. Individuals who consume white sugar, bread, pasta, and all other refined and processed carbohydrates tend to crave even more of these foods because of the "spike and crash" cycle, ultimately leading to weight gain. So that is where the whole issue lies. Many people blame their "staple" foods as being habitual.

In addition to being better for ensuring a balanced increase in blood sugar and stable insulin response, unrefined carbohydrates provide your body with more vitamins and minerals than refined carbohydrates because the refining process tends to remove those essential items. Unrefined carbohydrates include whole grains, such as brown rice, oatmeal, whole wheat, or bran; legumes, such as soybeans, peas, lentils, and peanuts; fruits, such as apples, strawberries, oranges, or grapes; and uncooked vegetables, like broccoli, carrots, and spinach.

The Glycemic Index Of Foods

The glycemic index of foods or GI refers to the categorization of foods, particularly sources of carbohydrates, on a three-point scale: low, medium, and high. Foods that cause an immediate rise in blood sugar are categorized as having a higher GI, whereas foods that increase the blood sugar at a gradual pace have a lower GI.

There are several diets out there that consider the GI as a way of determining the primary food nutrition groups to help people lose weight and keep it off for a long time. So it becomes extremely important for you to keep in mind what you eat when you begin with the lean muscle-building routine.

The following common foods fall under the low GI category: the majority of fruits and vegetables, the majority of dairy products, sweet potatoes, whole and unrefined grains, beans, and barley.

The following common foods fall under the high GI category: white bread, white rice, white pasta, peeled potatoes, corn flakes, ice cream, crispy rice cereals, cooked carrots, and sugars (excluding fructose).

The GI can be very helpful when you are creating your meal plan. For instance, it is best to eat foods under the high GI category immediately after an intense workout so that you boost and maximize the insulin response and regain muscle glycogen stores. Eating foods in the low GI category will help you lose weight, so concentrate on eating these while limiting your intake of high GI foods throughout the day. The chart below provides a sample of some commonly eaten foods:

Low GI (less than 55)	Apple, Broccoli, Cherries, Grapefruit, Orange, Pear, Tomatoes
Medium GI (56 to 69)	Banana, Brown Rice, Oatmeal, Popcorn, Sweet Potato, White Rice, Whole Wheat Bread
High GI (70 and up)	Bagel, Doughnuts, Rice Cakes, Pretzels, Watermelon, White Bread, White Potatoes

Now I'm sure your existing diet consists of all the foods mentioned in the last category. Don't worry; it won't remain that way for long, and by the time you are through with this book, you would have changed your food habits and will be on your way to attaining a lean and ripped body.

Counting Carbohydrates

For individuals who are starting an active lifestyle and trying to lose weight, your carbohydrate intake should fall within 100 to 150 grams each day. The sources of carbohydrates should primarily be vegetables and fruits. You can also eat small amounts of healthy starches, such as sweet potatoes and potatoes (with the skin), as well as whole grains, such as brown rice and oats.

Many people wonder if fruits are healthy, as they are sweet and have the capacity to add back fat to the body. In reality, fruits contain fructose, which is a more complex chemical than sucrose that is present in sugar. So if your body is exposed to both, it will take more effort for it to digest the former than the latter. In the process, it ends up burning more fat from the body. So don't think eating fruit is bad for you, unless you are eating extremely sweet fruits all throughout the day. However, you might have to exercise precaution if you have high levels of sugar in your body.

If you want to increase and speed up weight loss, you will need to limit your carbohydrate intake to the 50- to 100-gram range each day. This is also a healthy range for people who have Celiac disease or any other carbohydrate-sensitive issue. Concentrate on eating primarily vegetables and limiting fruit to one to three pieces per day, and avoid starchy carbs as much as possible.

To really rev up your metabolic rate, you should eat 20 to 50 grams of carbohydrates per day. If you eat less than 50 grams each day, the body will undergo a state of ketosis, which means that it will start to utilize the fat stores from your body as an energy source. You should only eat low GI carbohydrate vegetables, such as leafy greens, and trace carbohydrates from raw nuts, seeds, avocados, and berries. A word of caution: make sure to consult your doctor before making any drastic changes to your diet in order to avoid any health problems in the future.

Nicholas Bjorn

Chapter 3: Good Fats For Weight Loss

When we speak about obese people, we are referring to the fat that is stored in their bodies. It is no secret that Americans consume just so much junk that the fat they put into their bodies gets stored in theirs as their fat. The cumulative results are known, and the person might also find it tough to move about owing to his or her excess fat. However, it is possible for you to choose the kind of fat that you put into your body.

Not all fats are bad for you; eating the right kind of fat will help you lose weight and build lean muscle. But remember that fat contains 9 calories per gram, making it more than twice as dense as protein and carbohydrates (each of which is 4 calories per gram). Eating the right amount of healthy or good fats will help to keep you feeling full longer, thus assisting in the weight loss process.

The "healthy" fats are also needed by your body for managing your mood, achieving top brain function, fighting fatigue, and controlling weight. Your brain, for example, is almost 60% fat – that means that it needs fat in order to properly develop and function. These healthy fats can also help lower your cholesterol and the risk of heart disease, among other health benefits. The "unhealthy" fats, on the other hand, can raise your risk of heart disease and increase your cholesterol, as well as cause a variety of other negative health outcomes. This is why it is essential to understand which fats are good and which are bad, as well as to focus on eating the ones that will help your body.

There are four main types of fat found in today's diet of foods developed from plants and animals: monounsaturated, polyunsaturated, trans fats, and saturated fats.

Monounsaturated fats and polyunsaturated fats are considered to be the "good" fats, as they provide health benefits. Trans fats are definitively within the "bad" fats category, whereas saturated fats are still somewhat open to debate in the world of nutrition.

Omega-3 fatty acids are one of the most well-known types of polyunsaturated fats, and they provide a phenomenal amount of health benefits. These benefits include: preventing and reducing symptoms of ADHD, depression, and bipolar disorder; preventing memory loss and dementia; reducing the risk of stroke, heart disease, and cancer; easing the symptoms of joint pain, arthritis, and inflammatory skin conditions; and supporting a healthy and viable pregnancy.

The best sources for omega-3s are fish, such as salmon, herring, anchovies, oysters, and lake trout. For those who are vegetarian or do not eat fish for other reasons, there are other options: algae, walnuts, Brussels sprouts, spinach, flaxseed, and kale, to name a few. Given that there are restrictions for some people – including nursing mothers, pregnant women, and children under 12 – and the potential risk of mercury in fish, you may want to consider focusing on the non-fish sources, if possible. If you do really want to eat fish, check your local seafood advisories to see if the fish being caught locally are safe to eat, or choose fish that are lower in mercury, such as salmon, shrimp, and canned tuna.

There will be many websites and books out there that will tell you how no fat is good fat. But you need to understand that it is not possible for all fat to be bad, and there can be quite a lot of good ones as well. We look at those in detail and also examine what makes them healthier choices for those looking to lose excess body weight.

Understanding The Good Fats

It is easy to distinguish the good fats from the bad or unhealthy ones. Overall, as indicated above, the "good" fats will be monounsaturated and polyunsaturated fats, which include omega-3s. However, there are other factors that need to be considered when deciding on the specific foods that you will eat and determining whether they are providing good fats or bad fats. In addition to trans fats, and possibly saturated fats, unhealthy fats are those that have undergone chemical alteration or processing, especially from plant-based fat sources. Meat or dairy fat sources that come from farm-raised animals or mass production are also unhealthy.

On the other hand, plant-based fat sources that underwent minimal processing in order to retain most, if not all, of their natural state are classified as the good fats (for example extra virgin olive oil). Likewise, animal-based fat sources from free range, grass fed (organic farm) animals and wild game produce more healthy fats than unhealthy ones because the meat is leaner.

That is why several diets emphasize that grass-fed butter and other such fats should be used when dieting. It will help you lose weight faster, and you will not feel like you are dieting.

Good Fats From Plants

Unsaturated plant-based oils are the finest sources of healthy fats because they are composed of both monounsaturated fat and polyunsaturated fat. If your goal is to lose weight, choose:

- Avocados

- Almonds

- Macadamias

- Pecans

- Extra Virgin Olive Oil

These foods contain high amounts monounsaturated fats. As for polyunsaturated fats, the best sources come from foods that have not undergone processing, such as:

- Fish Oils

- Flax-Seed Oil

- Raw Seeds

- Nuts

It is important to have polyunsaturated fats in your diet, as your body is not able to produce these. They contain important omega-6 and omega-3 polyunsaturated fatty acids, also known as "essential fatty acids."

Here, we are referring to the butter that can be extracted from these ingredients. You can find these butters at any supermarket and use them for your everyday cooking. Just remember that you need to look for products that are genuine and not simply marked as healthy for commercial gains.

Many nutrition experts believe that processed oils from such sources as soybean, corn, sunflower, canola, safflower, and cottonseed should be avoided – despite being unsaturated – because they are manufactured through a more industrial, and less natural, process. Industrial processing is believed by some to have the potential to alter the "good" fatty acids into trans fats. If you are particularly concerned about the quality of the fats that you are putting into your body, then sticking with the products in the two lists above is the safest bet.

It is also important to remember that fats can go bad if damaged by heat, light, or oxygen. Keep in mind that polyunsaturated oils have to be refrigerated, and some unsaturated oils cannot be cooked at high heat as it will damage the fatty acids. If seeds, nuts, or oils smell or taste bitter – or more bitter than usual – then it is probably time to throw them out. You will want to make sure that you are eating the highest quality fats so that your body is able to get the maximum benefits.

Good Fats From Meat And Dairy

Eating grass-fed beef will nourish your body with the healthy fat called conjugated linoleic acid or CLA, as well as omega-3 fatty acids compared with eating grain-fed beef. As for fat from dairy, organic milk from grass-fed and free-range animals will provide you with healthy fat as well. Unfortunately, the same cannot be said of milk from pasteurized and homogenized milk. If you do not have access to "raw" or organic milk, the next best option would be to choose skim milk or coconut milk, almond milk, etc. These are the types of milk that vegans prefer, as they are strictly off dairy products. Again, you can buy these at your local departmental store, or look for them online.

Keep in mind that saturated fats are the primary type of fat found in red meat and dairy. While there is still some debate as to how good or bad saturated fats are for you, as mentioned earlier in this chapter, nutrition experts generally recommend that you limit your intake of saturated fats to less than 10% of your total calories for the day. Poultry is a good alternative for red meat because it will still give you some saturated fat while having a lower amount of saturated to unsaturated fats than red meat will provide.

If you are really determined to lose weight and build lean muscles in your body, then you will have to put in a little effort to cater to your dietary needs. If you think you can kick back and relax and expect to lose weight, then you are completely wrong. So don't look at these dietary changes as a tedious task, and consider them as your mission for your war against body fat.

Stay Away From Hydrogenated Oils

The worst kinds of fat are those labeled as "hydrogenated" or even "partially hydrogenated." These are highly toxic to the body because they cause arterial inflammation and, subsequently, heart disease and obesity.

Unfortunately, despite the fact that consuming these oils are detrimental to the body, they are widely available in restaurants and grocery stores because the hydrogenation process extends the shelf life of the oils, thus making them cheaper for wide consumption.

The rule of thumb for eating fat is to choose sources that underwent minimal processing and to control your portions. You do not have to concern yourself about whether they contain polyunsaturated, monounsaturated, or saturated fat because they will all be beneficial for your body as long as they are natural and organic. What you need to steer clear from as much as possible are processed foods and their trans fats.

What you will need to watch out for in particular are pre-packaged foods, including crackers, chips, candy, and microwavable popcorn, and commercially baked goods, such as cakes, cookies, muffins, and others. Unless they have specifically been made with alternative sources of oils, these types of products are likely to be quite high in trans fats and should be avoided whenever possible. Making your own is a great way to still enjoy the snack and ensure that you are limiting your intake of trans fats as much as possible.

If you need to cook with oil, choose butter, coconut oil, palm oil, or fine olive oil. Even though these are labeled as "saturated" fats, they still contain less free radicals and toxins once they are submitted to heat and light. However, it is highly advisable to choose non-frying cooking methods to minimize your use of oils, such as by baking, steaming, and boiling.

Most of these junk food chains use hydrogenated oil and butter to cook and fry. That is where your fat comes from. So don't eat these foods in excess, and in fact, don't eat them at all if you wish to remain healthy for long.

Try to include a small amount of healthy fats in your regular diet to maximize their benefits. Some food suggestions would be: a trail mix of raw nuts (such as walnuts, almonds, cashews, pecans and macadamias), seeds (such as sunflower, sesame, and flax seeds), and dark chocolate, yogurt, organic, or skim milk, as well as a teaspoonful of extra virgin olive oil with your salad or meat dish. Furthermore, you can replace mayonnaise with avocado (or guacamole), drink coconut milk or almond milk, eat organic peanut butter or almond butter, and take a fish oil supplement. These are not some things that you have occasionally (although that will also benefit your body). Instead, you need to try and include them in your diet as regularly as possible. Remember that you are trying to not just lose fats but convert them into lean muscles. Thus, you will need enough and more dietary help in order to supplement your exercise routine and attain a lean and ripped body at the earliest possible time.

Chapter 4: The Lowdown On Lean Protein

How many times have you heard someone saying that he or she is on an all-protein diet in order to build lean muscles? From wrestlers to actors, everybody prefers to go on a protein diet, as it is the one nutrient that is important for people to be able to start building strong and lean muscles that do not get burned away easily.

Protein is an essential macro-nutrient or building block that is known for repairing and creating muscle tissues. It is an essential part of fitness nutrition because it not only helps you lose weight but also promotes lean muscle growth. Now when you hear the saying "lean protein," it refers to protein sources that have low fat content.

Aside from building lean muscle mass, eating lean protein also makes you feel full for longer periods of time, which in turn will minimize your food consumption and help you lose weight.

In reality, if you are eating the required minimum amount of calories per day, then you are most likely consuming enough protein. But for building lean muscle mass, it is important to consider your sources of protein to ensure that this nutrient is coming with a well-balanced mixture of other nutritional elements.

Consuming protein helps your body burn more calories than fats or carbohydrates. Approximately 20% to 30% of the calories from proteins go toward the digestion process, while the range is between 5% and 15% for fats and carbohydrates. This is because protein is made up of amino acids, which are held together by very strong peptide bonds. Your body needs to be able to break down those bonds so that it can use the amino acids to repair tissues, move oxygen through your bloodstream, and form antibodies. In order to break those bonds, your digestion process has to work harder, which takes extra energy.

Remember, though, that just because you are getting more of your calories from protein instead of carbohydrates and fats does not mean that you can eat as many calories as you want. If you eat more calories, you will still gain weight, regardless of whether those calories are coming from protein or from other sources.

The best time to eat protein is about 30 to 45 minutes after your workout, regardless of whether you were doing cardio activities or strength training. During that window, your muscles are particularly focused on rebuilding and on repairing the micro-tears that form when you work out. If you give your body protein, that rebuilding and repairing process will work even better, making you less sore the day after and improving your lean muscle mass.

In order to get the most out of the protein that you are eating, choose a snack that has 12 to 14 grams of protein with a calorie amount of around 40% of what you burned during your workout. So for example, if you burned 300 calories on the elliptical, choose a snack that contains about 120 calories. Picking a snack that also contains some carbohydrates will help even more with muscle repair and energy replenishment.

Pick Your Protein

The major sources of lean protein are the following foods: fish, soy, poultry, eggs, mushrooms, beef, beans, peas, lentils, seitan, and dairy. You will notice that there are both vegetarian and nonvegetarian options here, and just because you fall into one of these categories does not mean you cannot attain lean muscles. While meat, poultry, eggs, fish, and dairy do contain all nine amino acids that we get from food – which is why they are often referred to as "complete proteins" – it is very possible to get all of the amino acids from plant-based foods if you eat a balanced variety of such foods. So stop making excuses, and start doing all the right things for your body. You need to keep in mind that having too much protein isn't a good thing, especially if you aren't working out. In fact, you only need between 40 and 50 grams of protein daily. If you aren't working out, this is a lot of protein and can actually do more harm than good. So, if you are working out, you need to make sure to get a good amount of protein in your system every day so you can effectively do your workouts. The protein will give you the energy you need to get through all the workouts and will keep you going beyond that. Let us look at each of these in detail and understand why they are important and beneficial for your body.

Fish

When it comes to meat, seafood is the best choice because it contains lower levels of saturated fat than beef and poultry. Many nutritionists prefer this and suggest it to their clients, as they think the body will fare better if they consume fish and go slow on other types of meats. Cold water fish, such as salmon, cod, herring, mackerel, and monkfish, should be on top of your list because they contain especially high levels of omega-3 polyunsaturated fatty acids and are quite low in calories, usually having 100 calories or less per a cooked portion of 3 ounces. These are also great for your heart, which means that you will prepare your body for intense workouts. Your immunity will also improve, and you will fall sick less often. You will have the chance to combat illnesses better, and your body will be able to undergo fitness training for longer periods of time.

Seafood is a very convenient protein source because, in addition to the benefits listed above, it also happens to contain all nine of the amino acids that our bodies need to get from food. That same 3-ounce cooked serving discussed above, which has 100 calories or less for certain types of fish, will also provide about one-third of the average daily recommended amount of protein.

Seafood is also a good source of protein because the protein it contains has less connective tissue than is found in poultry and red meats, so it is easier for your body to digest. For anyone who has stomach issues, particularly issues with digesting food, seafood can be an excellent option.

Take note that frying fish will remove most or all of its healthy fat content. Aim to have around 3 to 5 servings of fish for protein each week. You can decide to bake it and season it lightly, as well as use the leftovers for a salad.

Soy

Soy is a protein-rich food which, according to The Food and Drug Administration of the United States of America, can reduce the risk of heart diseases. Food based on soy is proven to have a small amount of saturated fats, which can be seen as a reason for the previously mentioned effect of soy food. Soy food provides the human body with magnesium and protein, and it helps in lowering cholesterol. Products made of soy, including edamame, tempeh, tofu, milk, nuts, and many others, are becoming more and more popular among people with healthy living habits, not just among vegetarians or vegans. Aside from being an important source of protein, soy is rich in fiber, vitamin B, and omega-3 fatty acids. Thus, it is a very healthy alternative for foods that contain large amounts of cholesterol and saturated fat.

If you are interested in introducing more soy into your diet but are not sure how to do so, it is actually quite easy: check out the vegetarian or "health food" section of your local grocery store. Today, there are vegetarian options for almost every kind of meat or dairy product, including veggie dogs and burgers, veggie ground round, soy milk and yogurt, and soy cheese. These products can usually be easily substituted into recipes rather than using the meat or dairy alternative. Just remember that soy products are not automatically healthy; as with any foods, check the nutritional label to make sure that the foods are low in cholesterol, saturated fat, added sugars, and salt.

While rare, some people will have digestion problems with soy products, and others may be allergic. If you are going to be introducing soy into your diet, it is recommended that you do it slowly, in small amounts, so that you are able to determine whether your body is going to have difficulty digesting it or if you are allergic.

Poultry

The second best choice for animal-based protein sources is chicken and turkey. However, both also contain high amounts of saturated fat, so choose the leanest cuts whenever possible. It also helps if you remove the skin before you eat it to further reduce your calories from fat. The healthiest ways to prepare poultry are by grilling, baking, or roasting. Although they are almost similar in taste, it is best for you to choose turkey over chicken. This will ensure that you are having a good helping of protein without any excess fat. It is also cheaper, and you will have a chance to consume it regularly. You can grill the meat after marinating it in something simple like lemon juice and fresh herbs, or you can also prepare spicy curries or fresh salads out of chicken and turkey meat. Just remember not to take away from fast food chains, and prepare everything at home by yourself, because the pre-prepared products tend to be very high in salt and added sugars, and possibly preservatives as well.

Eggs

Although eggs are known for their high cholesterol content, they are still a great source of lean protein because they cost less and have few calories. Eggs have been the go-to ingredients for wrestlers since time immemorial. There are several heavyweight champs who have lean muscles that go through 40 to 50 eggs a day. They need to consume it in order to build newer muscles and try and retain the old ones. Cooking eggs is almost effortless as well, and their versatility will allow you to sneak them into almost any dish possible. To minimize cholesterol intake, use more egg whites than the yolk. A good ratio would be to use three egg whites with one yolk. You can prepare an omelet with this ratio, and your protein intake through eggs is sorted. Eggs are also consumed by most vegetarians, so you don't have to worry about not getting enough protein if you are a vegetarian. Just boil some, slice it up, add to your fresh salad, and you are sorted.

Mushrooms

To the surprise of many, numerous nutritional attributes that are often found in different meat products or grains are also found in mushrooms. Mushrooms are proven to have a low amount of calories and fat, and they are cholesterol-free. Mushrooms are an important source of vitamin B, minerals, proteins, and beta-glucans. Another healthy attribute of the mushrooms is their anti-oxidant nature, along with the ability to strengthen the immune system. Similar to fruits and vegetables, mushrooms are proven to be gluten free, which makes them a great choice if you are on a gluten-free diet. As regards the amount of protein that mushrooms contain, 3.5 cups of mushrooms have 7 grams of protein. However, this amount of mushrooms has only 56 calories. The amount of protein is not high in comparison to some other products, such as meat, but with its low number of calories, mushrooms are proven to be one of the healthiest choices out there.

Beef

Many people are fond of eating red meat, and while red meat is a rich source of protein, it also contains high amounts of saturated fat. There are many who will stop eating red meat when trying to lose weight and build lean muscles in their bodies. In order to enjoy red meat without risking your health and forsaking your diet, choose the "round" and "loin" cuts or the "extra lean" ground beef, as these contain the least amount of fat. It is also best to trim off any visible fat right before you cook it to remove even more fat calories from your dish. These are the white areas on the meat. They give your meat its "marbled effect," and you will know to identify them as soon as you see them. Use a sharp knife to cut these parts out, and don't worry if they are too ingrained; a small amount won't harm you, and it is the large portions of the fat that you need to steer clear of.

Dairy

While dairy alone contains high amounts of fat, low-fat dairy, on the other hand, is a great source of lean protein. Dairy also contains calcium and vitamin D and has a low amount of saturated fat. Go ahead and add some Greek yogurt, low-fat cheese, and skim milk into your regular diet. You can also prepare your food at home if you think buying "diet" labeled dairy is expensive. All you have to do is to get rid of any cream from the dairy, and it will turn low fat. You can also make your yogurt low fat by getting rid of the foam that forms on top. The thicker that yogurt gets, the healthier it is for you. So try and make these at home as much as possible in order to help turn them into sustained parts of your diet.

Beans, Peas, and Lentils

Vegetarians rejoice over these plant-based sources of lean protein. They are extremely tasty and contain loads and loads of protein. In fact, just two small cups full of cooked lentils are enough for you to have the minimum dose of proteins required by your body. They also contain high amounts of fiber, which further helps keep you feeling full for longer periods of time compared to other foods. There are plenty of ways to prepare beans, peas, and lentils for a delicious meal. However, if you are planning to eat them frequently, make sure that the transition is gradual so that your digestive system can adapt, and you can avoid cramps, bloating, and gas. You can prepare a succotash out of the beans on alternate days, and lentils are versatile enough to be added to anything, including salads. Just cook them and add them to your soup, and as for peas, you can boil them and consume them as is.

Seitan

Another great choice for vegetarians looking for lean protein sources is seitan. With its origins in Asia, where it was used by monks, seitan's healthy effects are what make it popular among healthy eating people. This meal is made of the protein portion of wheat, and it contains 36 grams of protein per half cup. It can be mistaken for meat, and in many cases, vegetarians avoid it because the texture of seitan may resemble that of real meat. Whether it is braised in the oven, cooked in a pressure cooker, or baked, seitan is proven to be a great source of lean protein. For vegetarians who are looking for a quick but healthy bite, seitan can be a great choice because it is ideal for sandwiches. Moreover, seitan is also great for soups or any other type of meal that requires a meat substitute. Seitan is also great for barbecues, so even when you are with your friends having a barbecue, you are still able to eat healthily and maintain the protein intake at a needed rate.

Protein Portions

Your gender, age, and physical activity are three important factors that will help you determine the amount of protein that you should eat every day. For those who live a sedentary lifestyle (those who have less than 30 minutes of physical activity each day), the following recommendations are provided by the USDA:

For Men:

- 19 to 30 years old – 6.5 oz.

- 31 to 50 years old – 6 oz.

- 51 years old and above – 5.5 oz.

For Women:

- 19 to 30 years old – 5.5 oz.

- 31 to 50 years old – 5 oz.

- 51 years old and above – 5 oz.

Each ounce is roughly equivalent to 1 oz. of fish, meat, or poultry, 1 egg, 1 tablespoon of peanut or almond butter, 0.5 oz. of nuts or seeds, or half a cup of cooked beans.

As for those who live an active lifestyle (more than 30 minutes of exercise a day), it is generally recommended that you eat about 0.5 to 0.8 grams of protein for each pound of your body weight.

Chapter 5: Vegetarian Or Vegan?

The food you eat is incredibly important, but what if you don't want to eat meat? Being vegetarian or vegan doesn't mean that you can't lose weight or eat healthy; it just means there are different ways for you to go about doing that.

Veganism has a lot of benefits that some believe outweigh the things you'll be missing out on. For those of you who don't know, vegetarian and vegan are different. Vegetarians generally eat certain dairy products, like eggs, milk, and butter. Vegans, however, don't consume any animal products, meaning no dairy at all.

The reasons that you choose for going vegetarian or vegan are your own. Some want to try to stop animal cruelty in big industries, and they believe boycotting animal products is the best way to do so. Others find that going vegan is more beneficial for their body because of an ailment or sickness that they have. Still, others find that getting rid of animal products from their diet just makes their body feel better. Whatever reason you have, it matters.

Changing your lifestyle to vegan or vegetarian has tons of benefits. For example, many chronic illnesses can be avoided if you avoid a lot of the meat that you eat. Studies have shown that eating more fruits and vegetables actually reduces the risk of some cancers, heart disease, and Type-II Diabetes. Those who are at a higher risk of developing these diseases might consider changing their diet.

Different Kinds Of Vegetarian

You might be unaware, but there are a few different types of vegetarians. In fact, there are technically four different categories that vegetarians fall under.

Lacto-Ovo Vegetarians are the vegetarians most people think of. They will not eat any types of meat. Fish, poultry, and any products derived from animals will not be eaten unless it is part of the dairy family. Eggs and other dairy products are still eaten.

Lacto Vegetarians are almost identical to Lacto-Ovo vegetarians, but they won't eat eggs. They are free to consume any other dairy product, except for eggs. This is likely due to the fact that eggs can be hatched into baby chickens, but milk is just a byproduct of cows. They naturally produce this substance, and drinking milk isn't cutting off life.

Ovo Vegetarians won't eat any kinds of meat or dairy products, except for eggs. This could be because a person is lactose intolerant, or it could just be a personal preference. Eggs are jam-packed with protein and are easily one of the best ways to get protein as a vegetarian, along with nuts and other foods.

Partial Vegetarians have a little more leeway than others. There are also a few types of partial vegetarians. Generally, they pick and choose what meats they will and will not eat.

- **Peso-vegetarians (or pescatarians)** won't eat any meat except for fish. They usually also eat eggs and other dairy products, but meat and poultry are not on the menu.

- **Pollo-vegetarians** won't eat any meat or fish, but will gladly eat poultry. They will also usually eat eggs and other dairy products.

It's interesting that there are so many different types of vegetarians. For some people, going all the way and becoming a lacto-ovo vegetarian is too much. Having other options definitely helps. Also, if you want to take baby steps on your way to becoming a full vegetarian or even a vegan, there are a few ways to do that. You can slowly cut down the amount of meat you eat and then the types of meat. From there, you can slowly cut down on the others as well until you hit the desired end goal.

One Type Of Veganism

As for veganism, there's really only one type. All meat, dairy, and animal products are cut out of your diet. Some go even further and refuse to wear anything made from an animal, including wool, leather, and silk. They also will not use soaps or cosmetics that have animal products in them.

Being vegan can be very beneficial. You won't have to worry about needing any fiber in your diet, as vegan diets are typically high in fiber and many different vitamins and minerals. They are low in saturated fats, vitamin B12, vitamin D, calcium, and other things, some of which can be raised with supplements or finding specific foods with those things in them.

Properly Planned Diet

Having a properly planned out diet among both vegans and vegetarians is incredibly important. If you just start eating foods you know aren't meats but only eat certain ones every time, then you could easily lack certain things that your body needs. Any number of things could occur if that were to happen, so be sure to plan out a diet with your doctor or someone else who is a vegan or vegetarian.

The basics of a properly planned diet include having three full meals a day plus two snacks. These snacks are there to keep your blood sugar up and give you a boost in energy. If you are someone who generally skips breakfast, you should start eating a good breakfast. This can prevent you from eating the wrong foods later in the day.

Portion control is also very important. Just because you are eating a lot of healthy foods doesn't mean you can eat as much of that as you want, especially when trying to lose or maintain your weight.

Specific Nutrients

With any diet, there are some concerns that you won't get the required amount of a nutrient that your body needs. The same goes for vegetarians and vegans. There are plenty of nutrients that naturally occur in the foods that you are cutting out of your diet, which could lead to issues.

There are eight nutrients you should pay close attention to. If you find that the foods you eat aren't giving you the proper amount, look for other foods that contain these nutrients that you can add to your diet. If that isn't possible, talk to your doctor, and see if you should take a supplement.

- **Calcium**

This nutrient is incredibly important. It will strengthen your teeth and bones, something that becomes even more necessary the older you get. Most people think of the calcium that is in milk, but there is calcium in many different foods. Some of these foods might even surprise you.

There is a lot of calcium in dark greens, such as kale, broccoli, and other collard greens, as long as you eat a sufficient amount of them. Other calcium-enriched foods include soy milk, soy yogurt, tofu, juices, and cereal. They may not naturally have calcium, but calcium has been added in.

- **Vitamin D**

Just like calcium, vitamin D is important for your bone health. In fact, this vitamin actually helps you absorb calcium, which makes it even more important. This will help keep your immune system up and running, thus preventing you from getting various diseases that you might otherwise acquire.

The benefits of vitamin D go even further. There has been research that suggests vitamin D can actually help fight depression. It helps regulate your mood, which can then, in turn, alleviate some of your more severe symptoms. It can also help with anxiety, which often comes in conjunction with depression.

It can also help with weight loss. One study showed that people who were taking both a calcium supplement and a vitamin D supplement exhibited more weight loss than those who were taking a placebo pill. These two have an appetite-suppressing ability. If you have a deficiency in either of these, supplements can definitely help.

Vitamin D is naturally produced in your skin when it is exposed to sunlight. Obviously, don't stand out in the sun for an unsafe amount of time, but standing outside for 10 to 15 minutes without sunscreen can boost your body's vitamin D.

There are a few decent sources of vitamin D in foods. Salmon, for partial vegetarians, has a decent amount of vitamin D. Egg yolks also have some vitamin D. Orange juice, yogurt, and cereal are all fortified with vitamin D, making them not the best candidates for it, but they can still give you some of this vitamin.

- **Vitamin B-12**

Vitamin B-12 is crucial for your red blood cells. Having a deficiency of this vitamin can lead to anemia, which can cause a host of other issues. Unfortunately, for a vegan or vegetarian, it becomes a little more difficult to get this vitamin. This vitamin is also crucial for your nervous system health. It is crucial for keeping your hormones balanced and ensuring that the DNA synthesis in your body working at the full potential.

Unfortunately, many people with this deficiency have depression and anxiety, since their hormones are not as regulated as they should be. You can also become chronically stressed, which can take a huge toll on your body. Finding ways to boost your vitamin B-12 intake can be incredibly important.

There are many fish that have natural B-12 in them, but for vegans and vegetarians, there are alternatives. Breakfast cereals are fortified with this vitamin. Milk and yogurt also have some vitamin B-12. Hard boiled eggs are also a good choice to get more vitamin B-12. There are also some soy products fortified with this vitamin.

• **Protein**

There is a myth that has been going around for a long time about vegans and protein. Even though it's been proven wrong, many still believe that vegans and vegetarians, though to a lesser extent, don't get enough protein from the foods they eat. This actually isn't true. There are tons of alternatives to the protein in meat.

Protein is a vital part of your body. You need it in order for your body to repair any damaged tissues or cells. Your hair and nails are made up of mostly protein, so eating protein can help replenish those as well. It's a building block for most things in your body, including your bones, muscles, cartilage, and skin.

There are many alternate ways to get protein. Numerous vegetables, including spinach, French beans, peas, and kale, are packed with protein. If you're a fan of smoothies, try adding some hemp powder into them. This has plenty of protein and will help you get through the day. Different kinds of beans are also full of protein. They are part of the protein food group, so it makes sense that they would be a go-to ingredient in the world of protein.

Lentils are an interesting seed, but they are great and filled with protein. They can be added to rice dishes or veggie burgers to have that extra bit of protein. Quinoa is a wonderful and versatile food that can be used in so many different ways. Moreover, it has about 9 grams of protein a cup. Tofu is also a great idea when looking for protein-ridden foods.

Of course, various nuts are always filled with protein. Almonds and almond butter are great sources of protein. They can be added to any number of different meals to enhance them and give them an extra crunch. One last protein-filled food is chickpeas. They can be prepared in various ways, including hummus. Hummus is delicious, but you should try to use more actual chickpeas in various dishes. There is less sodium and more protein in chickpeas than in store-bought hummus.

- **Omega-3 Fatty Acids**

You might be wondering why you should want something with the word "fatty: in it. Make no mistake; omega-3 fatty acids are incredibly important to your diet. There are different types of omega-3s that do different things to help your body. They are ALA, EPA, and DHA.

ALA is mostly used to add energy to our cells, which keep us going. This fatty acid is also the building block for EPA and DHA. So, basically, if you don't have enough ALA, then you definitely won't have enough EPA and DHA. It works in conjunction with the others to help your body in various ways.

EPA helps with your inflammatory system, which acts when your body gets hurt. It acts as a natural anti-inflammatory agent, making it harder to become excessively inflamed, which can be damaging. Your body naturally reacts to damage by becoming inflamed, which then initiates cells from your immune system to start healing the damaged area. Some people have inflammation-related diseases, which can lead to higher rates of inflammation. EPA will help prevent that.

DHA specifically targets the nervous system, and the brain is surprisingly filled with DHA. This fatty acid makes up about 15% to 20% of the total fat in the brain, which is around 60% fat by weight. Research has shown that children who weren't exposed to a good amount of DHA tend to have slower neurological development or cognitive impairment. Adults can also be affected by the lack of DHA, with the chances of getting something like Parkinson's disease much higher than they might normally be.

All three of these omega-3s are important in some way to the natural functions of the body. So, is there anything else they could help? Depression, heart disease, rheumatoid arthritis, asthma, ADHD, and many other things can be alleviated with an increase in the consumption of omega-3 fatty acids. What kinds of foods should you be eating, especially if you don't eat meat?

There are a lot of foods with these in them. Flaxseed actually has the greatest amount of this particular nutrient out of anything else, making this a great thing to add to your vegan or vegetarian diet. Walnuts are a close second and are also an excellent choice in food. Beyond that, there are Brussels sprouts, cauliflower, soybeans, tofu, winter squash, broccoli, collard greens, spinach, and much more that are great for a vegan or vegetarian lifestyle.

- **Iron**

Many women in particular hear about how they need more iron in their diets. For everyone, iron is very important. Not having enough can lead to anemia, but having too much can lead to tissue damage. So, is it still really important? Iron is mainly used to help with oxygen transport. For women, menstruation will bring your iron levels way down.

As you menstruate, you release a mix of different things, including blood, which has iron in it. Girls who are just starting menstruation are at a higher risk of developing anemia because it's a whole new thing happening to their body. Making sure to eat iron-rich foods can help prevent anemia during menstruation for all women.

There are many foods that have a good amount of iron in them. For those who don't eat meat, there are dried beans, lentils, peas, fortified cereals, dark leafy greens, and whole-grain products. Along with this, you should eat plenty of foods with vitamin C. This will help your body better absorb the iron you're consuming.

- **Zinc**

Zinc is important for keeping your immune system working properly. It keeps your cells healthy and strong. There are also other health benefits that come from having a good amount of zinc in your body. This can help boost your athletic performance, giving you the energy that you need to complete these things. It can also help with fertility. Zinc is vital in maturing the egg and helping with fertilization.

Cancer is becoming very prevalent. A zinc deficiency has been found to lead to a multitude of different cancers, including that in the prostate, breast, colon, skin, lungs, ovaries, and leukemia. Having a good amount of zinc in your body can help prevent the occurrence of cancer in your body.

It's also crucial for your cardiovascular health. If you don't have enough zinc, it can lead to high cholesterol and a buildup of fat in your arteries, which can eventually lead to a heart attack. Zinc is also helpful in your insulin production, which can help prevent diabetes.

Just like iron, you don't want to have too much zinc in your body. It can lead to a ton of different things, including poor immune health and infertility. If you are thinking about taking zinc supplements, definitely talk to your doctor first. The foods you're eating might be giving you more than enough zinc.

Some foods to look at if you want to raise your zinc levels include nuts, soy products, whole grains, legumes, and yeast. Unfortunately, most vegetables aren't a good source of zinc, which is why many vegans and vegetarians have a lower zinc level. Therefore, if you really aren't getting the proper amount of zinc, talk to your doctor, and see if you should be taking a supplement.

- **Iodine**

This one may seem a little weird, but it's something your body needs. Having enough iodine in your system can lead to many benefits, some of which are mental and some are physical. Either way, this will help immensely with your overall health.

Having a good amount of iodine in your system can improve your cognitive abilities, which includes things like how you learn, how you complete tasks, and how you pay attention. Iodine also helps with your thyroid. Many people who have an iodine deficiency actually have an underactive thyroid. This can lead to weight gain because metabolism slows right down once your thyroid stops working hard.

For those of you with hormonal imbalance, maybe you don't have the right amount of iodine. Given that it helps regulate your thyroid, which also regulates your hormones, not having enough iodine can cause your hormones to start going haywire. Iodine can also add to your energy levels. If you've been feeling especially sluggish, then maybe you have low iodine levels.

Some people have thinning hair or hair that just doesn't grow very fast. Iodine can promote healthy hair growth. This doesn't mean you should get too much iodine in your system. Too much iodine is detrimental to your health, so you should definitely stick with a healthy amount of iodine. It's starting to be used as a type of antibiotic against certain pathogens. It's been shown to only kill off the bad bacteria and leave the good alone, which is something other antibiotics have been known to attack.

Iodine offers some protection against radiation. Some doctors use it on patients who've been exposed to too much radiation as a way to treat radiation poisoning. In the same vein, it offers some protection against cancer. The more regular your iodine levels are, the less likely you are to develop cancer. That doesn't mean you're completely immune, but the chances of getting cancer are reduced. Notably, iodine is crucial in preventing thyroid cancer. Given that iodine is so closely linked to your thyroid, it makes sense that having an iodine deficiency is more often seen in those with thyroid cancer than those without.

There are some foods that have a large amount of iodine. The vegan and vegetarian ones include dried seaweed, yogurt, eggs, strawberries, cranberries, and other sea vegetables. These foods, when eaten regularly, will keep your iodine levels in the appropriate zone.

Being vegan or vegetarian doesn't mean you're automatically deficient in the nutrients you need. It's easy to find natural ways to get certain nutrients. It doesn't matter what your diet is; there are always ways to find food alternatives to get the nutrients you need for a healthy body.

It Can't Slow You Down

Choosing a vegan or vegetarian lifestyle doesn't mean you'll lose out on things that you love. In fact, you might realize that this is the lifestyle you've been missing this whole time. If you have any medical condition, going vegan or vegetarian might be able to help. The focus on vegetables, fruits, and other healthy options might be exactly what your body needs to feel better.

You'll still be able to do everything that everyone else can do. You might not eat the same foods, but you will be able to work out, write, play, work, watch TV, and do everything else you can imagine. You might even notice that you have more energy than you did before to do those things. In the end, it's your choice, and you should stick with it.

Nicholas Bjorn

Chapter 6: Meal Frequency

At this point, you should fully be aware that weight loss highly depends on the amount of calories you consume versus the amount you burn off on a regular basis. You also know that lean protein is highly important for weight loss and for gaining lean muscle mass.

Another reason why you should include lean protein in each meal is the fact that it has the highest thermic effect among the three macro-nutrients, which means it provides the easiest calories to burn off.

Now the next question is this: how often should you eat in a day?

The Benefit Of Frequent Small Meals

Time and again, many fitness and nutrition experts stress the advantages of eating five to six small meals instead of two to three large meals each day. The main reason is that whenever you eat a small meal, your own body will help you expend a certain percentage of the calories during the digestion and absorption process.

On the other hand, if you eat large amounts of food at an infrequent and erratic rate, your metabolism will drop because the body will start to "preserve" its energy stores because it believes that you are starving in between meals. Even worse, with your body in this state, it will begin to break down the muscle tissues for energy use.

Large meals also have the effect of over-burdening your digestive system. Our bodies were designed to graze rather than to eat large amounts all at once, and when we introduce too much food into our system at a time, then our digestive processes are not able to keep up. In addition to a decrease in energy, this can also cause bloating and discomfort, which does not exactly encourage us to participate in physical activity.

There are many times when you'll go through the day and realize that you didn't stop and eat at any point. Generally, this means you'll end up having a big dinner because you're hungry. This does a lot more harm than good. If you eat small snacks throughout the day, it will actually help stop you from eating a huge meal. There will already be something in your stomach, so you won't be as hungry as you would if you hadn't eaten anything. This will cause you to have energy throughout the day and give you the ability to easily go and work out after your day at work.

Frequent small meals also help keep your blood sugar levels stable all day long. Because of this, insulin is not released as often, which keeps your insulin levels stable as well. Compare this with eating three large meals each day, which causes your blood sugar to increase instantly and then crash later on, thus triggering food cravings.

Adopting the approach of eating several small meals throughout the day can also help with your body's fatty acid levels: if you eat small amounts throughout the day, your fatty acid levels will remain much more stable, which gives your body a more consistent source of these vital components. In addition to ensuring a more consistent energy source, peaks and dips in fatty acids have been associated with a risk of heart disease, so avoiding those ups and downs will lower that risk.

Another advantage to eating smaller meals more frequently is that it tends to encourage people to eat a greater variety of foods, which in turns makes it more likely that they are ingesting all of the necessary vitamins and minerals. People who follow the "three square meals" routine, on the other hand, tend to repeat the same types of meals over and over again, which reduces the likelihood of getting all of the essential nutrients.

Thus, it is vital to adopt the five- to six-meal strategy in order to build lean muscles. There are several fitness experts and also celebrities who vouch for this theory's effectiveness in practically giving positive results. You might have your doubts initially, especially if someone says you need to eat two extra meals a day to lose weight, but trust me, you will understand how beneficial it is once you start on it.

The potential disadvantage of eating smaller meals more frequently is that you may be more likely to turn to pre-packaged snacks. Instead of buying your snacks throughout the day, try to make your own ahead of time. This will help you focus on healthier and more balanced snacks and avoid commercially prepared snacks that tend to be high in fat, salt, and sugar.

In order to maximize the benefits of the concept of frequent small meals, create a meal plan with meals that are spaced at about three hours apart. This means you should eat something as soon as you get up in the morning to pump up your metabolism instantly. There are many studies that show skipping breakfast causes weight gain. This is primarily caused by binge eating because the body has been "starved" earlier in the day.

To know how many calories you should consume per meal, simply divide the total number of calories that your body requires (or your target amount of calories) by 6. For example, if you plan to eat 2500 calories per day, then each of your six meals should be around 400 calories. For those who want to lose weight as quickly as possible, then it is recommended that you limit each meal to 300 to 600 calories. You may want to focus more of your calories on the first meal of the day and less on the last meal before bedtime, as your body requires additional energy in the morning to get going after a night's rest.

But remember, you are only splitting your entire day's meal into five or six portions while not having regular portions. You will end up getting fatter than you were in the beginning. So don't try and incorporate everything into your diet, and come up with a good meal plan that helps you attain and maintain a lean and muscular body.

A six-meal daily eating plan can vary drastically in content, and you can create one that incorporates many different foods that you enjoy. Here is a sample of what such a plan might look like.

Breakfast: 1 ½ cups of plain, non-fat yogurt with 1 cup of sliced berries, six almonds, and 1 cup of unsweetened whole-grain cereal, or one hard-boiled egg with two slices of whole-grain toast, ½ cup of orange juice, and 1 teaspoon of peanut butter (or another even healthier type of nut butter, such as almond butter).

Mid-morning Snack: whole wheat bagel with 1 ounce of low-fat cheese and a small apple, or a smoothie made with a small banana, ¼ an avocado, ¾ cup of fresh pineapple, and 1 cup of non-fat milk.

Lunch: turkey wrap with 2 ounces of turkey on a 6-inch, whole wheat tortilla with lettuce, mustard, 1 cup of vegetable soup, and an individually portioned-size container of non-fat yogurt. You could also try 3 ounces of grilled salmon with 2 cups of mixed greens, 3 non-fat whole-grain crackers, and 2 tablespoons of low-fat salad dressing.

Mid-afternoon Snack: a 6-inch whole-wheat pita with ¼ cup of hummus and 1 cup of sliced celery sticks and carrots. Or try a ¼ cup of raisins mixed with ¼ cup of unsalted mixed nuts.

Dinner: You could make some shrimp kebabs, with 3 ounces of shrimp and 1 cup of mixed peppers, onions, and mushrooms, served with 1 cup of mixed greens with 1 tablespoon of low-fat dressing and ½ cup of brown rice. Or you could prepare 3 ounces of beef tenderloin served with one small, plain baked potato and 1 cup of steamed broccoli.

Nighttime Snack: 1 ½ cups of unsweetened whole-grain cereal served with 1 cup of non-fat milk and a small banana, or 6 cups of air-popped popcorn (no butter!) mixed with 30 peanuts.

There are many foods that would fit in well with a meal plan that involves six small meals throughout the day, which means that you have the opportunity to create a varied and delicious meal plan for yourself. Keep in mind the various nutritional components that are important for you to be taking in on a daily basis and avoid pre-packaged, commercial products as much as possible. If you do all of this, you will be well on your way to achieving a daily nutritional plan that is delicious and nutritious and that will help you achieve lean muscle mass.

Nicholas Bjorn

Chapter 7: Fitness Nutrition Tips

Fitness nutrition is all about eating organic, whole foods and avoiding processed foods as much as possible. It highlights the importance of choosing your nutrition sources wisely by picking a lean protein, whole carbohydrates, and unprocessed monounsaturated and polyunsaturated fats so that you can lose weight and build lean muscles efficiently.

To help you transition from your old and unhealthy diet to an effective fitness-focused diet, here are valuable tips and habits that you can start implementing in your lifestyle immediately.

Create Meal Plans For The Whole Week

Make it a habit of planning your meals ahead of time, so that you will not run out of meal ideas and end up eating unhealthy foods. Keep a notebook where you can start jotting down your weekly meal plans, and create a template that will help keep your calories in check. It also helps to record all of your meal plans because you can use any set whenever you don't have the time to create a new one. It is important that you remain as prepared as possible in advance in order to remain on schedule every single day. When you are not prepared, you will be tempted to eat out; this will only harm your diet plan.

Another advantage of creating meal plans is that will encourage you to eat a wider variety of foods rather than just relying on what is already in your cupboards. If you come up with meal ideas ahead of time and go out and buy the necessary ingredients, you will be able to get more creative with your meal options. With greater variety in your diet, the more likely you are to get all of the vitamins and minerals that your body needs. It will also make you more likely to stick to the plan because you will not get bored as quickly or easily.

Hunt For Reliable Sources Of Nutritious Whole And Organic Foods In Your Area

Oftentimes, there are cheap and easily accessible food stores and markets in your area that you have not explored yet. On a free weekend, go out on an adventure to search for places that sell affordable yet high-quality fresh cold water fish, whole grains, and other carb sources and healthy fats. Make sure to take note of the prices and availability of these ingredients; you will find these notes to be very useful as you create your meal plan.

Your local farmer's market is a great place to start, as it will have a variety of foods for you to purchase and will also show you the local vendors from whom you can buy your food even when the farmer's market is not open or available. You might also want to consider local orchards and farms that often sell their products at their location or in local grocery stores.

In addition to helping you ensure that you are eating healthily and getting the necessary nutrients for your body, eating more locally will also benefit your community and the environment. It is a win-win situation for everyone involved.

Store Healthy, Whole Foods In Your Pantry And Throw Out Processed Foods Filled With Preservatives

At this very moment, open up a box, throw in all of the junk food and other processed meals in your home, and donate them to a local shelter. Next, create a list of your staple foods, including snacks, and then brainstorm for healthy alternatives to them. For instance, if you enjoy eating chocolate chip cookies every afternoon, you can replace them with whole wheat oatmeal cookies. If you are obsessed with soft drinks, replace them with soda water. If you love potato chips, substitute them with a bag of kale chips or sweet potato crisps.

There will also be a healthier and more natural alternative to your favorite snacks, which will be better sources of the essential vitamins and minerals and will almost certainly be lower in fats, sugars, and salt. Pre-packaged and commercially prepared foods are rarely the best option in terms of healthiness or nutrition, and the sooner that you remove these items from your pantry and your diet and start eating healthy and nutritious foods, the sooner that you will start to achieve your goal of increasing your lean muscle mass and being fit.

Be Conscious Of The Calorie Content Of Your Foods

Now that you know the impact of calories on your weight, you should start to become aware of the calorie content of the food that you eat. However, it might be inconvenient to whip out a calculator every time you have a meal, what you can do instead is to be more conscious of your portions and food choices. Try to imagine the foods in grams, and then remind yourself that proteins and carbohydrates have 4 calories per gram, whereas fats have 9 calories per gram. In this sense, you are more likely to choose baked salmon with a side of vegetables instead of a cheeseburger and some fries whenever you eat out.

There are many applications and programs that will make it easy for you to keep track of the calories that you are consuming and how many you are burning. These programs have databases that include the caloric content of most foods and the calories burned for different exercises, but you can also add the information manually most of the time. Once you start to keep track of the calories that you are eating and which foods are better or worse in terms of calories, you will be more inherently able to assess foods and determine whether or not they fit into your diet.

Stay Away From Refined Oils, High Fructose, And Trans Fats No Matter What

Whenever a food product includes the words "hydrogenated," "partially hydrogenated," "trans fats," and "fructose," stay away from it whenever possible. Do your best to prepare meals at home, and pack them for lunch instead of buying from a store or restaurant, as these places tend to have foods containing unhealthy oils (they are more cost-effective, after all). For snacks on the go, keep an apple, an orange, a banana, or a small bag of trail mix in your bag, and you will never have to eat fast foods.

Making your foods from scratch and using fresh ingredients – including fruits, vegetables, meats, and grains – will automatically ensure that you are avoiding these items because you will be aware of what you are putting into the dishes that you make or the snacks that you prepare. This will also allow you to be more accurate when you are keeping track of the calories that you ingest because you will be able to include the ingredients rather than guess at the calorie content of pre-packaged foods that do not always include a nutritional label.

This is another advantage of shopping at your local farmer's market; often, even the pre-packaged products sold at this type of location are a healthier alternative than the store-bought kind. Plus, you will be able to speak directly to the producers of the food to find out what ingredients are included, which will give you a better idea of the caloric content.

Have One Cheat Day Per Week

This must sound like a relief to many of you, but did you know that a cheat meal will actually help you with your weight loss goal?

While you do need to eat less than what you burn off every day in order to see significant weight loss, you will eventually hit a plateau wherein you cannot seem to drop any more weight.

Unfortunately, lowering your daily calorie intake even more will only cause you to lose the lean muscles that you have been working so hard to gain. This is caused by a hormone in the body called leptin. Low leptin levels will increase cortisol production and lead to muscle loss, a low metabolic rate, and an increase in appetite.

Now this is where your cheat day comes in. A "cheat day," which is the layman's term for infrequent overfeeding, is when you can eat whatever you want without counting calories. This will increase your leptin levels and bring them back to normal. During a typical cheat day, it is recommended that you add approximately 1000 calories more to your usual daily calorie limit. For example, if you have limited yourself to 1500 calories a day for 6 days a week, your cheat day should have 2500 calories. However, keep in mind that you should still stay away from soft drinks and other foods and beverages that are high in fructose because these pack a lot of calories without really giving you that satisfied feeling of eating.

You should also try and avoid eating trans fats on your cheat day as much as possible, because aside from the weight loss issue, trans fats can cause serious health problems. The important part of a cheat day for weight loss and muscle development is that you are not worrying as much about the amount of calories that you are eating, but you should still be paying attention to the types and quality of food that you are consuming if you really want to give your body the best health benefits possible.

Drink Tea To Help You Lose Weight

Hot tea, especially green, white, and oolong teas, is known to help promote weight loss because of the presence of caffeine, catechins, and polyphenols in them. These are substances that stimulate thermogenesis, which is a bodily process that converts fat to heat. This triggers an increased metabolic rate, enabling you to burn even more fat as you undergo physical activity. Furthermore, green and oolong teas help slow down the digestion of carbohydrates, thus keeping blood sugar levels stable and letting you absorb fewer calories with each meal. Include at least 3 cups of tea into your diet every day to maximize these benefits.

Always remember, though, that you need to keep track of anything that you are putting into your tea, either as a sweetener or in terms of milk products. If you are sweetening your tea with any kind of sugar, including honey, agave, or unrefined sugar, those do have a caloric content and will need to be included in your calorie count for the day. The same goes when you happen to add milk to your tea – remember to include the calories in your daily count. Each individual cup of tea may add minimal calories, depending on how much milk and/or sweetener that you use, but the calories can add up if you are having several cups per day.

Chapter 8: Calculating Your Daily Calorie Needs To Lose Weight

For our example on calculating your daily calorie needs, we are going to calculate calories and set a 10 lb weight loss goal using stats for the average American male:

Height: 69.3" OR 5 feet 9 inches

Weight: 195.5 lbs

Age: 25 years

Goal: Lose 10 lbs

And for the average American female:

Height: 63.8" or 5 feet 3.8 inches

Weight: 166.2 lbs

Age: 25 years

Goal: lose 10 lbs

BMR Formula

Harris–Benedict Formula

As a reminder, the BMR is the amount of energy required for a person's body to function. To calculate this, we use the current weight (195.5lbs), height in inches (69.3"), and age (25). Below are the calculations following the Harris–Benedict formula:

Male: 66 + (6.3 x body weight in pounds) + (12.9 x height in inches) − (6.8 x age in years)

= 66 + (6.3 x 195.5) + (12.9 x 69.3) - (6.8 x 25)

= 66 + 1,231.65 + 893.97 - 170

= 2,021.62 Calories Needed

Female: 655 + (4.3 x weight in pounds) + (4.7 x height in inches) − (4.7 x age in years)

= 655 + (4.3 x 166.2) + (4.7 x 63.8) − (4.7 x 25)

= 655 + 714.66 + 299.86 − 117.5

= 1552.02 Calories Needed

Mifflin St. Jeor Formula

Male: (10 x weight in kg) + (6.25 x height in cm) − (5 x age in years) + 5

= (10 x 88.7 kg) + (6.25 x 176) − (5 x 25) + 5

= 887 + 1100 − 125 + 5

= 1,867 Calories Needed

Female: (10 x weight in kg) + (6.25 x height in cm) − (5 x age in years) − 161

= (10 x 75.39) + (6.25 x 162.05) − (5 x 25) − 161

= 753.9 + 1012.81 − 125 − 161

= 1480.71 Calories Needed

Depending on which formula you choose to use – which is likely best determined by consulting with your doctor – the man would need to ingest between 1867 and 2021 calories per day, whereas the woman would need to ingest between 1480 and 1552 calories per day.

Physical Activity

For this example, we will keep it simple and focus on two main activities a person may complete in a given day: walking and exercising.

Walking: Based on a pedometer study completed in 2003, the average American walks 5,117 steps in a day, which is equal to 30 to 40 minutes of walking.

30 Minutes of walking = 228 Calories Burned for a 25-year-old male who weighs 195.5 pounds and is walking 4 miles per hour. For a 25-year-old female who weighs 166.2 pounds and is walking the same speed, she will burn 194 calories per hour.

Exercising: The general average amount of calories burned for exercises, such as fast walking, aerobics, fast biking, and running, in an hour is 419.

1 Hour of general exercise = 419 Calories Burned

Based on these two activities, the total number of calories required is:

Male: 228 + 419

= 647 Calories Needed

Female: 194 + 419

= 613 Calories Needed

Thermic Effect Of Food

As a reminder, the thermic effect of food is the amount of energy that the body utilizes in order to digest the food that you consumed. To calculate this, we use the total number of calories consumed within a day multiplied by 10 percent. For our sample, we use the same calories from the Harris–Benedict BMR calculation, 2,021.62 for the man or 1,552.02 for the woman, or the Mifflin St. Jeor calculation, 1,867 for the man or 1,480.71 for the woman.

Male:

2,022.62 x .10

= 202.26 Calories Needed

Or 1,867 x .10

= 1.87 Calories Needed

Female:

1,552.02 x .10

= 155.20 Calories Needed

Or 1,480.71 x .10

= 148.07 Calories Needed

Total Calories Required

Based on the three completed calculations, the total number of calories per day required in our example is BMR + Physical Activity + Thermic Effect of Food

Male:

2,021.62 + 647 + 202.16

= 2,747.78 Calories Needed

Or 1,867 + 647 + 187

= 2,701 Calories Needed

Female:

1,552.02 + 613 + 155.20

= 2,320.22 Calories Needed

Or 1,480.71 + 613 + 148.07

= 2,241.78

As you can see, after you consider the various calculations to be made, the numbers end up being quite close, regardless of the formula used. So the man would need to ingest somewhere around 2,700 to 2,750 calories per day in order to maintain his weight, whereas the woman would need to take in between 2,240 and 2,320 calories per day in order to maintain her weight.

Calorie Guideline To Lose Weight

For our example, the goal is to lose 10 lbs of body weight. As mentioned earlier, to achieve a 1lb weight loss, an additional 3,500 calories need to be burned in a week by reducing your portions, increasing your physical activity, or both; this is the only way to naturally change a pound of fat into energy and lose weight.

A simple guideline to follow is to reduce your calorie intake by at least 500 and no more than 1000 calories below your total daily required calories. Reducing your daily calorie intake by 500 each day for a week equates to a 1 lb loss in body weight per week. Therefore, to lose 10 lbs, calories will need to be reduced by 500 each day for 10 weeks.

Always keep in mind that even if you have done all of the proper calculations and are determining your required caloric intake to lose weight, your body does require a minimum amount of calories to carry out its basic functions. This is different from the amount of calories required to maintain your weight; this minimum amount is what your body absolutely cannot do without if it is to keep up with the necessary functions.

For women, that minimum amount is 1,200 calories; for men, it is 1,500 calories. So if, as a woman, your daily caloric intake would fall below 1,200 calories, if you were aiming to lose 1 lb per week, you should absolutely consult with your doctor before deciding to start a diet where you will be taking in less than that basic minimum amount.

If you do not make sure to eat the basic minimum requirement, your body will go into starvation mode, where it starts to break down your stored body fat for energy. Once it runs out of stored body fat, other body tissues will be broken down, and your bodily functions will start to break down.

If your body does not get the calories that it needs for its basic functions, you will start to experience nausea, fatigue, dizziness, and malnutrition. Diets of lower than 800 calories per day have been associated with the development of gallstones. In addition, when your body starts to break down bodily tissues for energy, which will include lean muscle mass, it will defeat the purpose of starting this reduced calorie diet in the first place. The disadvantages of reducing your caloric intake beyond the minimum requirement are far, far greater than the advantages.

Final Reminders

To lose weight as quickly as possible, each meal should be limited to between 300 and 600 calories. Carbohydrate intake should fall within 100 to 150 grams each day. To increase and speed up weight loss, carbohydrates can be limited to the 50- to 100-gram range reach day, or to really rev up your metabolic rate, go with 20 to 50 grams of carbohydrates per day. Those living an active lifestyle (more than 30 minutes of exercise a day) will need to eat about 0.5 to 0.8 grams of protein for each pound of body weight.

Nicholas Bjorn

Chapter 9: Best Upper Body Workouts For Lean Muscles

Remember that you need to supplement your diet with an exercise regime that will allow you to build lean muscles. You cannot rely on diet alone, as your body needs to work out in order to shape your muscles. For this, you can undertake upper body workouts that are beneficial to the muscles present in your chest, shoulders, forearms, biceps, triceps, and upper back.

The main muscles, or muscle groups, that you will want to focus on in this area are the deltoids, pectorals, trapezius (also known as traps), latissimus dorsi (also known as lats), triceps, and biceps. The deltoids and pectorals are found in your chest, the trapezius and lats in your upper and middle back, and the triceps and biceps, of course, in your arms.

We will look at exercises that target these specific areas and make sure that you attain a thorough burn each time. These exercises are a combination of equipment-based and non-equipment-based exercises, and you will reap the benefits of both once you start performing these.

There is also a segment on CrossFit training as it will help your body to indulge in some high-intensity interval training.

Let us start.

Nicholas Bjorn

Chest Exercises

Before you start with any of these, you need to warm up. For this, you can take up 30 minutes of cardio, such as running or jumping, and get your body warmed up to start with the exercise routines.

<u>Barbell Bench Press</u>

Barbell lifts allow you to generate the most power, which means that this bench press will let you move the most weight. Barbells are easier to control than dumbbells and thus serve as a great starting point if you are new to these kinds of exercises.

How to perform: Lie on the bench, and take hold of the barbell in the starting position. Lift the barbell, and bring it down slowly, while breathing in, until the bar touches in the middle of your chest. After pausing briefly, push the bar back to the starting position while breathing out.

Breathing is very important when doing this exercise. It gives your body enough energy to bring down and lift it back up. If you don't properly breathe, there's a good chance you could drop the bar on yourself.

Be sure to have a spotter, especially if this is your first time doing it or you are lifting a heavy weight. If there isn't anyone available, then make sure to lift a lower weight and not push it. Not having a spotter can cause a lot of issues, especially if you can't lift the weight back up. You should definitely know exactly how to do this workout before you attempt it. Not knowing how could result in you doing this incorrectly and hurting yourself or worse.

Dumbbell Bench Press

This exercise is great for all those trying to firm up their chest muscles. You will have positive results in no time. Dumbbells allow for more of a workout than barbells because dumbbells require each side of your body to work independently, which makes your stabilizer muscles work harder. This also means that not only does your chest get a workout, but so does your back, making this a great double-whammy workout.

How to perform: To perform this exercise, lie on the bench, and hold dumbbells (weight depends on your body type and strength) next to your chest. Next, turn them around slowly, such that your clenched fingers now face you. Slowly raise them upwards; you must feel the pressure on your chest. Hold for a couple of seconds before lowering it again and getting into the initial position.

Bent-Arm Barbell Pullovers

This exercise is especially great for building up your lats. It works the lats much better than the straight-arm barbell pullover because it works completely different muscles. This exercise still works some other muscles, like the pecs, triceps, and deltoids, but the main focus is on the lats.

How to perform: Lie on a flat bench, holding a barbell shoulder-width apart with your arms at a 90-degree angle from your body. Make sure that the barbell is held directly over your chest, with a bend in your arms. With your arms locked in the bent position, lower the weight slowly backward behind your head. Stop moving backward once you feel a stretch in your chest. Bring the barbell back up to the starting position using the same arching movement.

Dumbbell Chest Flyes

After doing this one a few times, you'll feel it in your chest. This exercise specifically strengthens your chest muscles along with your shoulders. You should do this one slowly, and make sure to not let the dumbbells touch at the top of the exercise. This not only adds to the exercise to make it harder, but it also forces you not to take too long of a pause.

How to perform: Lie on a flat bench with a dumbbell in each of your hands. Bring your arms up over you, shoulder-width apart, with your palms facing each other. Keeping a slight bend in your elbow, start to lower your arms in a wide arc to each side until you feel a stretching in your chest. Then bring your arms back up to the starting position, squeezing your chest muscles while you do it. Remember that this exercise's movement occurs through the shoulder joint, so keep the rest of your arm stationary.

What's great about this exercise is you can actually do it on either an inclined bench or a flat bench. This changes some of the muscles that you're working, so you can easily get two workouts just by changing the position of the bench.

Weighted Push Up

The push-up is a great exercise for your back and is one that will help in strengthening your chest muscles as well. Don't try this if you don't already have some upper body and back strength. There's a very good chance you could hurt yourself in the process. You have to modify the regular push up in order to make it beneficial for your chest, and here is how.

How to perform: Start by getting into the push-up plank position, and bring your hands closer, such that there is a 5-inch distance between them. Ask someone to place a weight on your upper back. Remember that the weight needs to be stable and something that puts equal pressure all over your back. Slowly lower your body and get perform the regular push up. Do as many reps as is comfortable.

It's pretty interesting that you can modify a regular push up to make it more of a muscle workout. It's a simple exercise that does require another person, but it can really send your muscle training above and beyond.

<u>Low Cable Crossover</u>

This exercise requires you to use a double cable pulley machine, which can be found in most gyms. It targets your deltoids and chest muscles at the same time, making it a great exercise to do when trying to build those muscles.

How to perform: Place the pulleys in the low position, and take one handle in each hand. Step forward so that the tension increases in the pulley. Turn your hands so that the palms face forward, keeping your hands below your waist and your arms straight. Bring your hands upward to the mid-line of your body while bending your arms slightly. At the highest point, your hands will be in front of your chest with your palms up. Then, bring your arms back down to the starting position.

Shoulder Exercises

Shoulder muscles need to be trained in order for you to have firm and good-looking shoulders. It can also help with any shoulder muscle pain that you may have. This could come from just having weak shoulders, which is why you would want to strengthen them in any way you could. Here are four exercises that will help you attain lean muscles in no time.

Seated Shoulder Press

This exercise looks extremely simple but gives your shoulders a good workout. It affects all the muscles in your shoulders, and you will start to feel the burn in no time. After doing this exercise consistently, you'll notice that you are more balanced in your upper body. You might even stand a little straighter because your shoulders have more muscle to them.

How to perform: Start by sitting on a chair, which should curve back a bit. Now hold dumbbells in both hands (weight of your choice), and hold them next to your shoulders. You need to have your fingers facing the other way. Now raise them up, and touch the two dumbbells together. Hold the position for a couple of seconds, and then the dumbbells them again, such that they are on par with your shoulder. Continue for 5 to 10 minutes or as per your convenience.

Battle Ropes

This exercise is best for those looking to strengthen their front deltoids. You will have strong deltoids if you perform these. It's also kind of fun to do, which is something that you should always look for in a workout. It's a good way to spice up your usual workouts and can be done at home if you wish.

How to perform: To start, buy yourself good quality battle ropes. Stand straight with the ropes in your hand and then squat, such that your butt is parallel to the floor. Now start moving the ropes up and down with full force. Remember to control the ropes; they should not control you. Do this for 5 to 10 minutes or as long as is comfortable.

Upright Barbell Row

The upright barbell row works quite a few muscles in your back, as well as your side and your deltoid. As you lift up, the muscle called *serratus anterior* is worked. It goes from your armpit down and is a good muscle to strengthen.

How to perform: Grab the barbell with an overhand grip, with your arms slightly less than shoulder width apart. Rest the bar on top of your thighs, with your arms extended and a very slight bend in your elbows. Keep your back straight. While exhaling, raise your elbows up and to the side, and use your shoulders to lift the bar. Keep the bar as close to your body as you can. Lift the bar until it almost reaches your chin, then lower the bar down slowly while inhaling. Remember that your elbows drive the motion in this exercise, and they should always be higher in the air than your forearms. Your torso must remain stationary for the whole exercise.

Side Lateral Raise

The side lateral raise is a great way to work your deltoids and other shoulder muscles. With strong shoulders comes less chances of hurting yourself when carrying heavy objects or doing anything that requires some shoulder movement. This can easily be done at home if you have a few dumbbells sitting around.

How to perform: Stand straight with the one dumbbell in each hand and your arms at your side, palms facing in. While exhaling, lift the dumbbells to your side while keeping a slight bend in your elbows and your hands tilted slightly forward. Keep raising your arms until they are parallel to the floor. Pause for a second, and then lower the dumbbells back to the starting position while inhaling.

Forearm Exercises

The forearm is a difficult area to train, and most people don't concentrate on it. But you need to consider each and every part of your body when you choose to build lean muscles. You might not realize it, but having strong forearms means you'll have a stronger grip. This is especially important in the law enforcement field, as those without a strong grip could easily lose their lives if they can't hold on to a suspect. It's also important for working out, because a stronger grip means you'll be able to hold on to weights much better. Not to mention that your forearms are the first thing many people see when they look at your arms, so you want them to look good. Let us look at a couple of effective forearm exercises that will help you build lean muscles in no time.

<u>Plate Pinch</u>

This is probably the best forearm exercise for you as it affects the forearm and helps you attain toned forearms without much effort. Be sure to start off with a lower weight, and slowly make your way up as you do this more and more. You don't want to hurt yourself right when you start to make a difference in your forearm strength.

How to perform: Start by holding two pinch plates that have been joined together. You can choose the weight that is apt for you. You can add more if you need to have a better burn. Hold it for 30 seconds, and then move to the other arm. Do three sets. It is best to do this after your shoulder exercises.

Barbell Hold

Performing the barbell hold is a great way to train your forearm muscles. Given that you have to focus on holding it for as long as possible, gravity plays a huge part, making this a very effective forearm exercise. Here is how you can do it.

How to perform: Start by choosing a weight of your choice. The barbell needs to have a thick rod for easy grip. Now stand in front of it, lift it from the stand, lower it back down, and allow your arms to stay normal. Hold for 30 seconds, and place it back. Do three reps.

Farmers Walk

This seems like a super simple workout. All you do is hold some weights in your hands and walk around. You shouldn't do it for longer than a minute, but even something like 30 seconds will be a pretty good exercise. Of course, you need to make sure to have dumbbells that you are able to carry around for an extended period of time. Don't start with 45 pounds if you have little to no arm muscle, as you'll only end up hurting yourself.

How to perform: Pick up a dumbbell in each hand. With a straight back and your arms hanging down at your side, keep the dumbbells at your side. Then start to walk back and forth. This exercise seems to be very simple, but what makes it a great workout is the time that you put into it: it is recommended to start with 30 seconds and work your way up. Your forearms and other muscles will start to burn faster than you might think.

Biceps Exercises

For all that who not aware of what biceps are, they are the three muscles that lie between the shoulders and the elbows. This is a problem area for many people as they do not lift heavy weights on a regular basis and end up having a lot of fat built up. These are also the muscles that are commonly used when lifting heavy objects. If you don't have strong biceps, you might not be able to carry all that much and definitely not for long periods of time. Here are two effective exercises to help you attain toned biceps.

Chin Ups

Chin ups are exercises that you perform in order to firm up your bicep muscles, and this particular exercise affects all three of the muscles involved, viz. the biceps brachia, the brachialis, and the brachioradialis. These are similar to pull ups, but they have many differences. A pull up has a much wider grip than a chin up and also uses different muscles. Generally, with a pull up, you want to get up above the bar a little higher than just your chin. However, with a chin up, you need only touch your chin to the bar in order to succeed. These are great to quickly build up your biceps.

How to perform: Start by finding a tall enough bar that helps you pull yourself up fully. Now hold it tightly by keeping a 12-inch gap between your hands, and pull yourself up such that your chin touches the bar. Lower yourself down again. One rule of thumb is to always follow the 2:2 motion for your biceps. So for every 2 seconds you spend in the chin-up position, you need to spend 2 seconds in the chin down position. Repeat as many times as is comfortable.

Barbell Curls

This exercise is mainly for the biceps brachia, but you will feel the burn in your forearms and the rest of your biceps as well. This is a very effective exercise and can make a difference in all of your arm rather than just your biceps, which makes this a great exercise.

How to perform: Start by choosing a heavy enough barbell. Now stand straight, and hold it in your hands. Don't hold it like you normally do; your thumbs should be on top. Now pull it up by curling your arms, and make sure the rod touches your chin. Hold the upward pose for 2 seconds and the downward pose for 2 seconds. Continue for as long as is comfortable.

Dumbbell Curls

This exercise is similar to barbell curls, but of course uses dumbbells instead of a barbell. Try to keep the dumbbells level as you bring them up and then back down. This will make this exercise the most effective. It's a great alternative to the barbell curl if you would rather use dumbbells.

How to perform: Standing straight, take a dumbbell in each hand at arm's length. With your elbows kept close to your torso, rotate the palms of your hands until they face forward. Keep your upper arms fixed, and curl the weight upward, contracting your biceps. Make sure to exhale during this part. Keep raising the weights until the dumbbells are aligned with your shoulder, and you have fully contracted your biceps. Hold this position for a brief pause, then while inhaling slowly, lower the dumbbells back down.

Triceps Exercises

Triceps are the muscles on the back of your arms between your shoulder and elbow. The triceps are a set of three muscles that are known as the lateral head, the medial head, and the long head. You must perform exercises that will affect all three in order to build lean triceps. Having stronger triceps means you'll have more shoulder stability, which in turn makes it so you are able to do a lot more. Let us look at a couple of the triceps exercises that will give you the best results.

Dips

Dips are great for both men and women looking to work on their triceps. Having toned triceps helps your hands look muscular and healthy. You will not need any equipment to perform these, and they can be easily done at home. However, there are pieces of equipment at a gym that will allow you to do dips. This is generally attached to a machine where you can also do pull ups. Often, this machine has a seat to help assist you with pull ups and dips, but it can be moved out of the way if you don't need assistance.

How to perform: Start by finding two parallel benches with a little gap between them or just a low enough chair. Start by sitting on the chair, placing your hands next to you, and gripping the edge tightly. Now get your butt off of it, and lower it below the level of the chair. Now go down and up, down and up, and make sure you are using your triceps to assist you in the motion. To add leverage to it, you can place your legs on top of the bench in front of you or another chair.

Overhead Extensions

Overhead extensions are best for your entire triceps region. It is important for you to develop the "horseshoe region" in order for your triceps to look good. Be sure to have a good grip on the dumbbells, or you might drop them. Moreover, make sure you don't hit your head as you do these, as that could result in a very bad injury if hit hard enough. You can affect these by performing overhead extensions, and here is how you can do it.

How to perform: Start by holding a dumbbell in your hand (weight of your choice), and stand straight. You must do this one hand at a time. Now lift it up and over your head. Hold the position for a couple of seconds and release. Do as many times as needed, and you need to feel a proper burn in your triceps.

Seated Dumbbell Press

This can be a very effective triceps workout that can build your muscle beyond where you thought it could be. If you mix this with a few others, your triceps will be more than strong enough.

How to perform: Sit on a bench that has some back support, and place the dumbbells upright on top of your thighs. Using your thighs for support, place one dumbbell in each hand, and lift each dumbbell up one at a time until it reaches shoulder height. Turn your wrists so that your palms face forward. This will be your starting position. While exhaling, push the dumbbells up so that they touch over your head. Pause and then bring the dumbbells down to starting position while inhaling.

This exercise does not have to be performed on a bench with back support, but it is recommended, especially for people who experience lower back issues.

Upper Back Exercises

The upper back muscles are slightly hard to train, and not many perform exercises that are apt for this area. Thus, many people ignore this area because they think of their arms, chest, and core first. The upper back is incredibly important. If you have a stronger upper back, you'll be able to have better posture, and you'll be less likely to injure yourself. Your back is what keeps you upright in the first place, so neglecting it doesn't seem like a very smart idea. You don't need to put all of your focus on the upper back, but you should give it some focus to make sure it's strong enough for your needs. You can choose the following for your regime:

Barbell Pull Over

The barbell pullover is quite basic but affects your upper lats, which are in your upper back. This exercise is incredibly useful, especially since you can use a barbell. Barbells, in many ways, are actually more efficient and easier to control than dumbbells are. You don't need to focus as much on having everything parallel, as all of the weight is on a single bar, rather than you holding two separate things. Here is how you can use this exercise to your advantage.

How to perform: Start by lying on the bench. Now hold a barbell in your hand and over your face. Now push it backward over your head, such that it is lower than your head level. Hold for a couple of seconds, and then lift it back up over your head.

Arm Pull Down

This is another exercise that is great for your upper back and works on the entire region to give you well-toned muscles. This specifically targets the lats and will make your back much stronger. This is a great exercise to do when you find that other exercises are more of arm exercises and don't help your back, even if they should help a little. This one, however, will make it so you have very strong lats.

How to perform: Start by standing in front of the pull-down machine. You can also make yourself one by tying ropes to dumbbells and pulling them over a high rod. Now stand straight, and jut your chest out. Pull the weights down. and make sure your upper back is feeling the burn. You can do around 15 reps and four sets.

CrossFit Training Regime

The CrossFit training regime is a good way for you to exercise all the muscles in your body, and the short bursts give it a good burn. You can try out these upper body CrossFit routines to have a mean and ripped upper body. These workouts are meant to be challenging and varied. Your body won't know what hit it after every exercise. Of course, doing different exercises is the best way to lose weight and get fit. If you do the same exercise for too long, then you'll be stuck at a plateau and won't know how to continue on from that. Doing the CrossFit training regime might just be one of the best things you could ever do, as long as you're up for the challenge.

You will always start out doing a warm up. This is simply meant to get your body moving and warmed up so it will be a lot more difficult to hurt yourself while doing something in the program. The best thing about this program is that it's meant to take your body and make it able to do anything. It won't be just strong or just fast, but it will have an even mix of every possibility. These classes will be incredibly intense, but they are more than worth it in the long run, so don't be afraid to go out and try it.

Many of the workouts are given names, and one of the examples we look at is called **LYNNE**.

For this, you perform bench press and pull ups alternately. You do five rounds, and each one should contain maximum repetitions. These max repetitions are up to you, and you must do them until you feel the burn in your chest, arms, and entire upper body. You can try and outdo yourself every time, but don't push yourself too hard. You can take a 5-minute break between the rounds.

You should ideally be done with this in 30 minutes.

FRAN

Fran is an easier workout routine if you are unable to do Lynne.

This follows a pattern where you alternate between thrusters and pull-ups. Here is the Fran pattern for you:

21 thrusters, followed by 21 pull ups

Then 15 thrusters, followed by 15 pull ups

Then 9 thrusters, followed by 9 pull ups

You can take a 2-minute break between each and be done with it within 10 to 15 minutes.

Remember that these are performed in short bursts with rest allowed only after the set workout is done. If you are feeling too tired, then don't continue, and try to reduce the work out time.

There are tons of different workouts within the CrossFit training regime. If you find a class and go to it, you'll likely do many different sets of workouts every time you go. Maybe you'll find a few that you'll easily be able to do at home or at a gym. Then, you can do it there instead. If you want to continue in the class, you're more than welcome to do that as well. Nothing is impossible with the CrossFit training regime.

Chapter 10: Best Lower Body Workouts For Lean Muscles

Now that we looked at the upper body exercises in the previous chapter, we will shift our focus on lower body exercises. The lower body, specifically the legs, is sometimes an afterthought for someone who's trying to look his or her best. It absolutely shouldn't be. Your core and your legs are the foundation to your body. If your legs and core are both weak, you'll have a lot more trouble doing things than others might. These exercises will help you build up the muscles you need and start on the right path.

Abs Exercises

Abs refer to the abdominal muscles, which can be toned to look like small square blocks. Most people looking to build a lean body are also looking to build strong abs. In general, this is the part of the body you hear most people talk about when getting into shape. Everyone marvels at the abs. There is a stereotype that people are truly fit when they have a six pack, which is the name that's usually given to abs. You can be fit without having noticeable abs, but that doesn't mean you can ignore the abs.

Having abs is incredibly important to the overall structure of your body. Given that it is in the core of your body, having abs makes it much easier to do certain things and also makes your body much more balanced and structured, as long as the rest of you is as well. Although it is slightly tough to chisel out washboard abs, it is easy to firm them up and get rid of belly fat by performing these ab exercises.

Crunches

There are several crunches that are building blocks for firm abs. Performing crunches daily can help in building lean and strong abs. Crunches are great because they can literally be done anywhere that you can lay down. If you travel a lot, you can still do crunches every day. They don't require a gym. There are many types of crunches, but we will look at the three main ones that aid in fixing your belly fat problem.

Basic Crunch

This is the most basic crunch that you can perform to firm up your abs. You need to perform this daily if you wish to strip your belly off of fat and firm up both your upper and lower abs. This crunch is super easy to do, and anyone can do this crunch. All you need to be ready is some space on the ground. This crunch is great for people who don't really have any abs. It's a great place to start building your ab muscles. However, if you already have some established abs, it might be best if you skip doing this crunch. It will likely do little to nothing for you.

How to perform: Start by lying on the floor. Next, bend your legs and put your hands behind your head. Now slowly put enough pressure on your upper torso to lift it up. You must remain there for 1 second and then go back to neutral position. Do 50 to 60 (or lesser) reps, depending on your level of comfort. If you are finding it tough to do this, then you can hold out your hands instead of placing them behind your head.

Twist Crunch

The twist crunch is great for your lower abs, which are generally hard to reach. You can perform this to chisel out your lower abs, as well as your laterals. This one might be a little harder for some people, as there is a twisting element to it. Anyone who has any hip issues may want to avoid this one and focus on something else instead.

How to perform: Start by lying on the floor and placing your legs over a high platform like the bench or stool. Place your hands behind your head and raise yourself up to twist to one side. Go back to neutral, and repeat on the other side. Then go back to the right side. If you wish to add an extra level of difficulty, then place a weight on your chest. You can perform this on alternate days. Do 50 to 60 reps (or lesser), depending on your level of comfort.

Bicycle Crunch

The bicycle crunch is a variation of the twist crunch. It is meant to help you strengthen your abs. This ab workout definitely works more of your body than just your abs. You'll get a leg workout, along with an ab workout, which can be very satisfying. Let us look at how it is performed.

How to perform: You need to lie down on your back and bend your legs. Bring your knees towards your chest while lifting your upper torso. Now place your hands behind your head, and while turning to the right, straighten your left leg. While turning to your left, straighten your right leg, and so on. You should really feel the burn in your ab area. You can do 10 repetitions and 5 sets.

Leg Raises

Leg raises are great for your lower body. They will tone and give your lower body a good structure. This workout is one of the best non-machine ab workouts there are. It really forces you to tighten your abs to be able to not let your legs hit the ground or stop moving. You should do this workout slow, as going quickly won't help you in any way. This is a great one to do on a yoga mat, if you own one. The extra bit of support might be very helpful. Here is how you can perform this exercise.

How to perform: Start by lying down and lifting your legs 90 degrees in the air. You can place your palms under your butt and slowly lower your legs, but don't let your legs hit the ground. Raise them again and then lower again. Continue until you feel a good burn in your abs.

Circle Raises

This is a more complex ab workout than some of the others on this list. Your legs will be in the air for a while, so you need to have a strong core to keep it up. This would be best done after you begin to form abs. This way, you'll be able to up the difficulty of your ab workout, giving you the ability to grow your ab muscles even more.

How to perform: Start in the same position as before. Now lift both legs, and lower them slightly. Keeping the right leg stable, turn the left leg clockwise and then anti-clockwise. Repeat it with your other leg. You can then join both legs and do the same. You can do 5 reps for each leg.

¾ Sit-Ups

This is another more difficult ab workout. This one can be hard to understand at first, but once you get the hang of it, you'll likely be able to do this one without any issues.

How to perform: Lie on the floor, and with your legs bent at the knees, secure your feet. Put your hands on the side of or behind your head. Starting with your back flat on the ground, flex your spine and hips, and raise your torso to your knees. At the height of the contraction, your upper body should be perpendicular to the ground. Start moving back toward the ground, but only go ¾ of the way down.

Air Bike

This exercise sounds fun, but it is a lot of work and will do wonders for your abs. You need to keep in mind that if you pedal too quickly, you will lose any of the work that you tried to do. It will feel like you did barely anything. Keep a constant pace that isn't too crazy fast or too slow. You need your abs to get somewhat of a workout, and they won't get them if you're too fast or too slow. Make sure to tighten your ab muscles while you do this as well; otherwise, you won't be doing much of anything.

How to perform: Lying flat on the floor with your lower back against the ground, put your hands beside your head. Lift your shoulders so that you are in the crunch position. Bring your knees up so that your lower legs are parallel to the floor, and your knees are perpendicular to the floor. Now imitate a cycling motion: kick forward with your right leg and bring your left knee toward you, while bringing your right elbow forward to your left knee. Go back to the starting position, and then repeat on the opposite side. Continue alternating until you have performed the recommended number of repetitions for each side (not total!).

Barbell Side Bend

This can be a very satisfying exercise. It will require your body to move back and forth, giving your abs a side workout, which is something they don't get very often. People with hip or lower back problems should probably stay away from this exercise. There's a good chance it will only cause further injury, which is not something you want.

How to perform: Standing up straight, hold a barbell on the back of your shoulder, just below your neck. Make sure that your feet are shoulder-width apart. Keeping your head up and your back straight, bend right at the waist as far as you can while inhaling. Hold that position for a second, and then return to the starting position while exhaling. Repeat the movement to the left side.

You should not try this exercise if you have lower back problems, as it can cause further damage.

Barbell Ab Rollout

This exercise is quite challenging and should only be tried by people who have strong and healthy backs. If you have lower back problems, avoid this exercise. For less advanced athletes, you can try this exercise on your knees rather than standing on your feet. If you are having any trouble understanding how to do this one, find someone who knows how to do it or find any video of how to do it. This way, you'll know for sure whether you're doing it right or not.

How to perform: Starting in a push-up position, grab on to a barbell that is lying on the floor in front of you. Keeping an arch in your back, lift up your hips, and roll the barbell toward your feet while exhaling. Keep your abs tight, your back slightly arched at all times, and your arms perpendicular to the floor. Pause at the peak of the contraction, with the barbell as close to your feet as you can get it. Then, roll the barbell back to the starting position while you inhale.

Thigh Exercises

Thighs are a problem for several people. A lot of fat can get stored there, and normal exercises don't help in eliminating this fat. The idea is to perform exercises that will target this area of the body. The thighs are particularly a hotspot of fat in women. Once a woman goes through puberty, it's pretty easy for her to get a buildup of fat in that area depending on the foods she eats. For men, the stomach area is a higher concern with fat than the thighs, although men can still have their thighs as the main problem area. Here are exercises that help in targeting thigh fat.

Jump Squats

Jump squats are meant to help people tighten their thigh muscles. These can be very intense, but you need to make sure to fully come down before jumping again. You can easily lose your balance with this exercise, which is why it's crucial to center yourself before you jump again. You can easily lose a lot of thigh fat by doing this exercise in conjunction with other exercises.

How to perform: Splay your legs a bit, and crouch down. Next, jump up with your arms in the air, and jump back down. You need to land with a crouch. Repeat it until you feel your thighs strengthen and burn. Continue until your thighs are fully firm. You can jump up and down 15 times and gradually increase it to 20 and so on. This exercise might look simple, but it is not. You need to put in effort to jump up and land on your feet fully. You must stand on your toes and jump to make it easy for yourself. If it is too strenuous on your feet, then you can choose to stand and simply squat in the same place. Then get up and go down again.

Walk Squats with Weight

This is a great thigh workout that gives your body a nice amount of stretch. It's always good when a workout can actually stretch you out along with helping you build muscle or lose some weight. This doesn't require you to hold a weight, but it does give it a bit more of a challenge, so you might want to do that.

How to perform: Start by placing one foot in front while pushing the other backward to squat. You can hold a weight in your hand if you like. Repeat with the other foot, and keep walking forward. You need to keep the motion going until you feel stiffness in your thighs.

Ball Leg Lifts

This exercise requires an exercise ball, which is an excellent way to add a bit of a challenge to the standard basic exercises. The extra work that is required to keep the ball in place uses multiple muscle groups, in addition to the focus muscle group of the exercise that you are doing. This particular exercise will work your thighs, particularly your inner thighs, as well as your core. Make sure to be relatively cautious with this exercise. You don't want to overextend something or hurt yourself, so be sure to take it easy and know exactly what you are doing before you attempt it.

How to perform: Lying on your side on the floor with your arms crossed in front of you, place the exercise ball between your feet. Slowly lift the ball toward the ceiling using your butt and hips only. Pause at the top, then lower the ball to the floor. This is one repetition. This exercise works well if you complete 3 sets of 15 reps.

If you are uncomfortable with your arms crossed in front of you while lying on your side, you can try bending your bottom elbow and resting your head on your hand.

<u>Glider Side Lunge</u>

While this exercise officially calls for using an exercise disc designed for this type of activity, in reality, you can use a paper towel on a wood or tile floor or the lid of a plastic container on a carpet. This exercise focuses on one side in particular, but it really works that one side. Given that you are sliding with this one, make sure you are careful. You don't want to over slide or slide too fast, as that could result in you falling or injuring yourself. Keep the object you're sliding on steady as you go into the squat.

How to perform: Standing with your feet several inches apart, place your right food on the disc (or lid, paper towel, etc.). Make a fist with one of your hands, and then cup the other hand over it. Make sure to keep your hands in front of your chest while doing this exercise, as it will help you to stay balanced. Put your weight on your left leg, and then bend your left knee and squat while sliding your right foot out to the side. Then straighten your left leg, and slide the right foot back into the center. Do 3 sets of 10 reps with each leg.

<u>Gate Swing With Cross</u>

This exercise provides a deep inner-thigh stretch and will tone your quads, glutes, and your inner and outer thighs. There is a lot of stuff going on in this exercise, even if it seems rather simple. It's a pretty intense exercise that requires you to really keep your balance and take care of yourself. You could easily mess up and hurt yourself, so start out slow. As you feel more comfortable, go faster. Of course, as your muscles grow, you'll be able to do this exercise more effectively and make the most of it. Just make sure not to go into it too fast.

How to perform: With your feet in a wide stance and your toes pointed outward, bend your knees and lower into a squat. Use your hands to push your knees further apart, which will deepen the stretch. Pushing off of your knees to get leverage, jump your right leg in front of your left leg so that you end up standing cross-legged. Then immediately jump back out into a wide squat, with your hands at your knees. Repeat with your left leg going in front of your right leg. For sets and repetitions, just repeat this exercise with the right and left leg alternating for at least 40 seconds.

Lower Leg Exercises

Lower legs have calf muscles that need to be trained and shaped. You need to exercise and train your calves into attaining a toned look. Your calf muscles are incredibly important to your body. There are many risks associated with weak calf muscles, especially for athletes. You are more likely to tear your Achilles tendon, which is crucial for your leg to work properly. For non-athletes, there are still risks associated with weak calf muscles, including poor blood flow and not having a full range of motion in your ankle. Let us look at exercises that help you tone your calf muscles.

Leg Raise With Weights

Leg raises are the best way to tone your calf muscles. They will target the exact muscles that need to be toned. All this exercise requires is a weight and some sort of stool or chair with a proper height. It can be easy to do this incorrectly, so make sure you are careful with keeping everything straight and controlled. Let us look at how you can perform these to tone your calf muscles.

How to perform: Choose weights that are appropriate for your body. Now turn away from the stool, and place your leg on it by lifting it backward. Hold the weight in your hand, squat forward, and then alternate with the other leg. Continue alternating until you feel a burn in your calves. Don't stop until you are completely tired.

Similarly, you can do dumbbell step ups. For this, hold the dumbbell in your hand, and place one foot on the step. Alternate with your other leg, but don't step too fast. Continue until you feel a burn in your calves.

<u>Seated Calf Raise</u>

This exercise can be done at home or at the gym using the calf exercise machine. Given that it is a versatile workout, it is much easier to do. This calf exercise not only strengthens the calf muscles but also stretches out the front of your ankles. You might be a little sore afterwards, but it is definitely worth it. Of course, if you have any ankle problems, make sure you can do this exercise safely before attempting it.

How to perform: If at home, sit on a sturdy chair with your feet flat on the floor and your knees directly over your feet. Lean forward, and place your hands on your thighs near your knees, pushing down to add resistance. Press the balls of your feet down slowly while raising your heels as high as you can. Once you have raised your heels as high as possible, slowly lower them again.

At the gym, sit on the calf press machine, and place the balls of your feet on the platform. Use the machine to release the weight onto your calves, lower your heels as far as you to get the weight at its lower starting point, then press the balls of your feet down, and raise your heels as high as possible.

<u>Barbell Squats</u>

Barbells are used to help the body feel greater weight while you squat to tone your muscles. This can be considered an advanced exercise, and you must take it up only if you have been exercising for a long time and have already dealt with all the fat in these areas. This is almost solely a muscle-building exercise because of what you're doing. The weight from the barbell is pushing down on your entire body, so when you go back up, you need to push against not only the weight, but gravity as well. This is what makes this exercise so successful. This can also be done on a machine where the barbell is attached. That will make this and any other barbell exercises much safer, as there are clips on the barbell to stop it if necessary.

How to perform: Choose an appropriate barbell. Now hold it behind your shoulder. You can ask someone to hand it to you. Balance yourself, and squat down. You need to feel the burn in your calves and other muscles in your body.

Hip Exercises

Hip exercises are meant to strengthen your hips and the muscles around it. These exercises are especially important for women to take up, as they need to maintain strong hips. Some of these exercises will also be very helpful for people who have had a hip injury or surgery, as these will help strengthen the hips and prevent the issue from happening again. Even if you are someone who hasn't had any hip injuries, it is always good to keep your hip muscles well-formed and strong to prevent any potential future injuries.

<u>Hip Lifts</u>

Hip lifts are a great choice if you have a lot of fat accumulated there and need to get rid of the majority of it. It is best that you perform these if you have a strong back, and steer clear if you have back problems. This will also help strengthen the abs, given that you need to have something that will keep your torso and leg in the air.

How to perform: Start by lying on your back. Now bend your legs. Lift your right leg in the air, and balance your left leg with the heel. You must raise your lower torso as well. Do this 10 times, and keep alternating your legs.

If you would like something a little easier to start with, you can ignore lifting your leg. Lay on your back with your legs bent 90 degrees. Lay your hands on either side of your hips and slowly lift your hips up, making them in line with your knees. Hold this for a few seconds, and lower your body back down, but don't touch the ground. Repeat this for a total of 10 times and 3 sets. Just like with the other exercises here, this will utilize your hips and your abs, making it a great workout.

<u>Lateral Squats</u>

Lateral squats are slightly easier, and you can perform these even if you have a back problem. These will also effectively deal with your hip muscles. This is one of those exercises that are deceptively easy. You might not think you are doing a whole lot, but it's really working your hips and strengthening them, which is exactly what you want. Just make sure to not push too far to either side. You don't want to tear anything in your hips.

How to perform: Start by standing straight. Now put your hands out in front, and hold them parallel to the floor. Squat a little, and shift all your weight to one side. This can be your left. Maintain your balance while doing so. Now shift to the other side, and keep alternating. You will feel both your hips and your hands tighten. Continue until you feel comfortable.

Standing Side Kick

This exercise targets your glutes, quads, and inner thighs, as well as your outer hips. This is a great exercise that can also stretch you out. If you can't quite make it to be parallel with your hip, that's okay. As you progress, you might be able to make it there, as this exercise both stretches and strengthens the hips. This will initially be a lot easier for people who already have a lot of flexibility.

How to perform: Stand with your feet hip-width apart, and place your hands on your hips. Slowly extend your right leg out to the side, eventually getting to hip height (or as close as you can get). Make sure that your inner thigh is kept parallel to the floor. Hold the leg at the peak for 1 count, then lower back to the floor. The raising and lowering should each take 3 counts. Do 15 repetitions, then switch to the left side and do 15 repetitions on that side.

Side Jump

This is a fun little exercise. If you wanted and had kids, you could do this with them and make it a sort of game. Maybe you could try to psych them out and jump when they least expect it. This is one of those exercises that is easy to do, even when you have kids running around. It might be a little hard at first, but once you get the hang of it, it will be a great exercise to strengthen your hips.

How to perform: Stand with your hands on your hips and feet slightly less than shoulder-width apart. Hop 3 feet to the left and land on your left foot with your left knee slightly bent. Then bring your right foot down onto the floor. Repeat the exercise to the right. Continue the repetitions until you have done 15 on each side.

Butt Exercises

Butt muscles are easy to train if you get into the right positions. Your butt is a pretty important part of your body. If you've ever noticed that it gets uncomfortable when you're sitting, it likely means that your glutes aren't very strong. If that's the case, getting your glutes into a muscular state will definitely help. Moreover, it will make your body look much more balanced. If you have a strong upper body, you should definitely have a strong butt as well if you want your body to look proportional. Let us look at some of the exercises that you can take up to train your butt.

Kick Back Squats

This exercise helps your butt stretch out and contract. You will feel really good once you are done with this exercise. This will not only help you get your butt into the state you want it to be in, but it will also give you a nice cardio workout along with your toning workouts.

How to perform: Start by standing straight. Now bend forward by putting both your hands in front and lifting back your right leg. Hold this pose for a couple of seconds. Return to neutral position, and jump up and down into a squat. Now bend forward and lift your leg. Continue doing this until your butt feels firm.

Backward Leg Raises

This exercise is meant to help you tone your butt. This is a great exercise that will definitely tone your butt to the look and feel you want. It relies on you using your core and making sure that you have good balance, as you don't want to fall over. Let us look at how you can perform this exercise.

How to perform: Start by sitting on the floor on all fours. Have your palms in front of you and your legs next to each other. Now look straight and upwards, and lift your right leg high in the air. Point at the sky with your foot, and raise it as much as possible. Hold the pose and feel your butt muscle stretching. Now bring your leg back down. Repeat with your other leg. Do 10 repetitions and 2 sets on each leg.

If you want a bit more balance in this exercise, experiment with holding out the arm opposite of the leg you have raised up in front of you. Try to keep your leg and arm steady, and use your core muscles to help keep yourself straight. Hold this pose for a few seconds before bringing both back down and switching to your other side. This will also help strengthen your hip muscles.

Pigeon Pose

This is a simple exercise that will help in toning your muscles. You need to perform this after performing the other two in order to add leverage to your work out. This is a great exercise to help stretch and tone your body. The more exercises you do for both stretching and toning, the better. It will help keep you loose in the middle of your workout and prevent you from getting too tight, which will only inhibit your movements.

How to perform: Start by sitting on the floor. Now fold your right leg, and place it in front of you. Push your left leg backward. You can stop here or continue to bend forward, and stretch your hands out in front of you fully. Now get up and alternate your legs. You should feel your butt completely stretching out. This should firm up your butt, and you must feel a good burn.

CrossFit Training

Just like CrossFit for the upper body, you can take up CrossFit for the lower body. CrossFit exercises are some of the most intense workouts you'll likely ever do, but they are incredibly rewarding. Let us look at some workouts for you.

<u>Jack Squat</u> – jumping up in the air and landing with a squat

<u>Lunge</u> – bending forward with one foot in front and the other sliding backward

<u>Clock Lunge</u> – performing regular back and forth lunges and alternating with side lunges

<u>Single Leg Deadlift</u> – bending forward to touch toes while raising alternate legs backward

<u>Twisting Squat Jump</u> – jumping up and turning mid-air to land on the floor facing the opposite direction

<u>Scissor Squat</u> – jumping up and landing in a lunge with alternate legs

Do this within 5 minutes, if possible, with 5 repetitions of each.

If you feel like your body is getting used to it, then you can choose to continue with it for a longer period of time. There are many other workouts for this, which you can easily find online or by going to a class. The classes for CrossFit training are incredibly intense, but they can be incredibly beneficial. This will allow you to try new things that are varied with every workout that you do. Your body will easily transform in front of your eyes as long as you go to these classes consistently. Once or twice a week is a great way to start, and you should definitely also workout outside of class times. This way, you'll be able to stay in shape and be ready for the next class. They really are intense, but these classes are held in many places all around the world, so it shouldn't be too hard to find one near you.

These make up the various lower body exercises that you can perform in order to tone and strengthen the muscles present in your lower body. Doing these exercises in conjunction with other exercises will make your body look the way you have always wanted it to look. You will have toned muscles and a figure that makes you happy, which is all that truly matters. As long as you feel healthy and happy with your body, then you are all set.

Chapter 11: Alternative Exercise Choices For Lean Muscles

You must remember that you do not always have to indulge in cardio exercises to maintain a lean body. You can also take up less intense exercises, such as Pilates and yoga, to attain lean muscles. Both of these workouts are wonderful and are more beneficial than some people believe. Many people look at yoga and think that it's girly and that it's not something that could possibly help them. Others look at it and think that there's no way they'd ever be able to do the poses that others can. Both of these beliefs are wrong. Yoga is incredibly beneficial to not only women, but also to men. It is beneficial to anyone who wants to get in shape, lose weight, or become more flexible and balanced in their life. All of these are good reasons to give yoga a try. If you want to try something else, Pilates is also incredibly useful. Pilates aims to do very similar things to what yoga does, but in very different ways. That doesn't make it any better or worse, but it is definitely interesting to look at both of them. Here are the best exercises from each for you to try out.

Best Pilates Moves

This set is best for women who cannot hit the gym and have only a little time to exercise. You can use this set to achieve a lean upper body. Pilates is a way to get a great workout in not too much time, because it focuses on developing good posture, flexibility, balance, and strength all at the same time. It's not quite a full body workout, but it definitely works a lot on your body. It works your legs, your core, your glutes, and your back. The only one it doesn't work is your arms, but with the other benefits that Pilates has, it doesn't matter. You can work your arms doing different things after your Pilates workout.

It's a low impact exercise – one that anyone can do. It focuses on working your muscles strongly, but that doesn't mean it can't also be gentle. If you're at home and just really can't make it to the gym, doing this workout can be a great thing.

All you need to perform this is a resistance band that you can buy from any sports equipment shop or order online.

There are 4 exercises that you can perform to achieve a good burn. Let us look at these 4 in detail. Remember that the quality of the moves is more important than quantity: make sure that each repetition is done as cleanly and strongly as possible, rather than focusing on the number of repetitions. For beginners, focus on moving slowly and using the correct form; for those who are more advanced, you can try holding 1 to 2 lb dumbbells while you perform the moves.

Exercise 1: Start by standing with your feet spread out but your heels touching. Hold the resistance band in your hand. Now raise your heels and stretch the band over your head and then push it behind your head. You need to completely stretch each and every possible muscle in your body while doing so. Hold the position for a couple of seconds, and then release. You can do 15 repetitions and 3 sets of this exercise. You can increase it if you think it is possible for you to push your body more.

Exercise 2: Next, sit on the floor or the mat. Maintain a straight back, and splay your legs slightly. Place the resistance band across the arches below your feet and hold it stretched out. Now bend your knees slightly, and bend forward to try and touch your chest to your knees. You need to push the resistance band backward in doing so. Maintain this pose for 5 seconds and release. You can do 15 repetitions and 5 sets of this exercise.

Exercise 3: Lie on your back, and place the resistance band on an anchor that is placed 1 foot above the ground. Now lift your legs in the air and bend them at the knees, such that your lower leg is parallel to the floor. Hold the resistance band, and pull it down while lifting your head, neck, and shoulder. This will help the muscles in your head, neck, and shoulders burn. You can do 15 repetitions and 3 sets of this.

Exercise 4: Sit on the floor, and stretch your legs out. Wrap the resistance band around the arches below your feet. Now tilt back a little, and lift your legs up. Don't lose balance and fall back; the idea is to balance yourself on your butt. Now bend at the knees, and have your lower legs parallel to the floor. Stretch the resistance band, and try and bring your hands over your shoulders. You can do 15 repetitions and 3 sets of this and increase the number if your body is capable of taking on more.

If you do not have an exercise band and do not want to invest in one, or if you want to see whether Pilates is for you before you purchase an exercise band, you can try the following moves at home using only a workout mat or some other similar surface.

Exercise 1: The Pilates Curl

Lie on the floor face up, with your knees bent and your feet flat on the floor. Have your arms at your sides. While exhaling, curl your chin to your chest and bring your shoulders completely off the mat. Hold this position for 1 breath, then lower back down slowly. Lift from your breastbone to make sure that you are engaging your abs; this will also help you to avoid injuring your neck.

Exercise 2: The Hundred

Lie on the floor face up, and bring your knees toward your chest. Lift your head, neck, and shoulders off of the mat, and stretch your hands out to your sides with your palms facing the floor. Extend your legs out at a 45-degree angle, with your heels together and toes apart (this is called the Pilates stance). Pump your arms up and down while breathing in and out through your nose for 5 counts each. Repeat the move for 10 sets.

Exercise 3: The Roll-Up

To do this move, lie face up on the floor with your arms extended toward the ceiling. While exhaling, curl your chin down to your chest and roll up to a sitting position with your arms reaching toward your feet. While inhaling, reverse and roll back down to the floor one vertebrae at a time. Make sure that you move slowly and smoothly, and that there is no forward jerking or lunging.

Exercise 4: The Ball Roll

Sit on your mat with your knees drawn toward your chest and your arms wrapped around your legs. Rock back onto your tailbone, with your feet just a few inches above the mat. Inhale and then roll backward until your shoulder blades touch the floor. Exhale and roll forward to the starting position. Use your abdominal muscles to control your momentum, and make sure that you stop your movement forward before your feet touch the mat.

You can do these exercises on a daily basis, and try to do them twice a day for the best results.

Best Yoga Poses

Yoga is an ancient Indian exercise program that has been performed for hundreds of years. The poses that yoga prescribes are capable of massaging your body from the inside. All of the poses that you do in yoga will benefit you in some way. There are poses that relax you after having done some more intense poses, but even those will stretch you out and let your body take in everything it had just done. Yoga also has many benefits outside of the obvious. It can truly be a life-changing workout that can not only make your body stronger, but also relax you. Let us look at these poses in detail.

Pose 1: Downward Facing Dog

This pose is meant to help your back, abs, and legs have a good burn. You can start by lying flat with your face to the ground. Now use your palms to push your upper body upwards and your feet to push your lower body upwards. You, along with the floor, need to form a triangle. Now look in front, and raise your left leg high in the air. Push as much as you can. Hold the pose for 2 seconds and return the leg back to the ground. Now raise your right leg and hold for 2 seconds before returning it back. You can do 10 reps and 2 sets.

Pose 2: Surya Namaskar

The Surya Namaskar is a pose that helps the entire body and requires you to perform intense exercises successively. There are 12 poses in all, and they are as follows:

Start by standing straight and joining your hands to do Namaste. Now lift your hands and push them upwards and backward, and do the same with your back and neck. Now quickly bend and touch your toes. Bend down and push your left leg backward, and perform a forward lunge. Push your right leg back, and get into the upper plank position. Now quickly lie on the floor and look up. Push yourself up to attain the downward facing dog neutral pose. Now perform the forward lunge with the left leg forward, and quickly get up to touch your toes. Bend backward, and come back to the Namaste position again. Do 5 sets.

Pose 3: Wheel Pose

The wheel pose will stretch out your spine completely and work on your abs to firm them up.

To perform this pose, start by lying face down on the floor. Now bring your heels towards your butt and raise your head, neck, and shoulders. Bend your hands backward to grab your feet, and pull them towards your bent head. Remain in this pose for 5 seconds, and then go to the neutral position. You can do 5 sets of this pose.

Pose 4: Warrior Pose

To perform the warrior pose, start by standing straight with your hands on your side and legs joined. Now place your right leg forward, such that your thighs are parallel to the floor. Push your left leg backward simultaneously. Now join your hands, and lift them above your head. You can stare at your palms. Hold for a couple of seconds, and go back to the neutral position. Repeat this 5 times.

Pose 5: Bridge Stand

To perform the bridge pose, lie flat on your back. Now bend your legs, and place your heels as close to your butt as possible. Lift your lower torso and balance your upper body with your head, neck, and shoulder. Join your hands between the gap that is created under your lower back. Hold for a few seconds and release. Do this 10 times.

For beginners, you can make the pose easier by placing a stack of pillows under your tailbone.

Pose 6: Mountain Pose

To perform the mountain pose, put your feet together and stand tall. Relax your shoulders and make sure that your weight is distributed evenly through the soles of your feet. Start with your arms at your sides, then take a deep breath and lift your arms over your head, palms facing each other and arms straight. Reach toward the sky with your fingertips.

Pose 7: Tree Pose

To perform the tree pose, start by standing with your arms at your sides. Stand with all of your weight on your left leg, and be sure to keep your hips facing forward throughout the entire movement. Pull your right foot up to rest on the inner part of your left thigh. Once you feel that you have balance, bring your hands in front of you in a prayer position, with your palms together. While inhaling, extend your arms over your shoulders, palms separated but still facing each other. Stay in this position for 30 seconds, then lower your arms and repeat the pose on the opposite side.

This position can be difficult at first. For beginners or those with difficulties balancing, you can bring your right foot to the inside of your left ankle, rather than your left thigh, and keep your toes on the floor. This will help with balance. As you improve in doing this pose and develop better balance, you can move your foot to the inside of your left calf, then eventually up to your thigh.

Pose 8: Triangle Pose

For the triangle pose, stand with your feet about 36 inches apart, with the toes on your right foot turned out to 90 degrees and the toes on your left foot turned out to 45 degrees. Extend your arms out to your sides, and then bend over your right leg. Let your right hand touch the floor or rest on your right leg just above or below your knee. Extend your left hand's fingertips toward the ceiling. Look up to the ceiling and hold the pose for 5 breaths. Stand and repeat the pose on the opposite side.

Pose 9: Seated Twist

This pose stretches your shoulders, back, and hips, as well as increases your circulation and strengthens your abdominal muscles and your obliques. To perform the seated twist, sit on the floor with your legs extended in front of you. Cross your right foot over the outside of your left thigh, and bend your left knee. Keep your right knee pointed up to the ceiling. Move your left elbow on the outside of your right knee, and keep your right hand flat on the floor behind you. Twist to the right as far as you can, moving from your abdomen. Make sure to keep both sides of your butt on the floor. Stay in this position for 1 minute, then switch sides and repeat the pose.

For beginners, you can make this position easier by keeping your bottom leg straight and placing both of your hands on your raised knee. If you find that your lower back is rounding forward, sit on a folded blanket.

Pose 10: Cobra Pose

For the cobra pose, lie on the floor face down, thumbs placed directly under your shoulders. Extend your legs out, with the tops of your feet flat on the floor. Tighten your pelvic muscles, and pull your hips downward, squeezing your glutes. Press your shoulders down toward the floor and away from your ears. Push down with your thumbs and index fingers while raising your chest toward the wall in front of you. Relax and repeat the pose 4 more times.

Pose 11: Pigeon Pose

This pose works on your piriformis, which is one of your deep gluteal muscles. To perform the pigeon pose, start in a full push-up position with your palms aligned under your shoulders. Place your left knee on the floor near your shoulder, with your left heel by your right hip. Lower down onto your forearms, and bring your right leg down with the top of your right foot on the floor. Keep your chest lifted to the wall in front of you, but stay looking down. Pull your stomach in toward your spine, and tighten your pelvic floor muscles while contracting the right side of your glutes. Curl your right toes under while pressing the ball of your foot into the floor, pushing through the heel. Bend your knee to the floor and release. Do 5 repetitions in total, then switch sides and repeat.

For more advanced or more flexible practitioners, instead of keeping your chest lifted toward the wall in front of you, you can bring your chest down to the floor and extend your arms in front of you. This will provide a deeper stretch and will work the target muscles more.

You can perform these poses twice a day to receive their full benefits.

Chapter 12: Six Of The Best Lean Muscle-Building Recipes

In this chapter, we look at meals that are loaded with protein, which will help your body attain maximum protein intake.

Easy Egg Breakfast

Ingredients:

- 5 egg whites
- 1 egg yolk
- 1 garlic clove, minced
- 2 teaspoons mustard
- 2 teaspoons cayenne pepper
- Salt to taste
- 2 teaspoons olive oil
- 2 teaspoons fresh basil, chopped
- 2 teaspoons fresh oregano, chopped
- Fresh coriander leaves, chopped

Method:

- Start by placing the egg whites in a bowl and beating until firm.
- Add in the yolk, and beat until well combined.
- Now add the crushed garlic, mustard, cayenne pepper, salt, basil, and oregano, and give it all a good mix.
- Heat a pan, and add in a little oil.
- Add in the egg mix.
- Allow it to scramble before making a large omelet out of it.

- Place it on a serving plate, and sprinkle with coriander leaves on top to serve.
- You can add in tomatoes and chopped avocado if you wish to consume this meal as a weight loss recipe.

Cucumber Tartine

This recipe is an easy, quick snack that provides a lot of nutrition. It is a great choice for a mid-afternoon snack. It does not require any cooking, so you can pack the ingredients separately and put them together when you are ready to eat, ensuring that it is as fresh as possible.

Ingredients:

- 2 tablespoons part-skim ricotta cheese
- 2 tablespoons crumbled feta cheese
- 1 slice whole grain bread, toasted
- 9 to 12 cucumber slices, very thin
- Sea salt or truffle salt

Method:

- Mix the cheese together in a small dish.
- Spread the cheese mixture on the toast.
- Layer the cucumber slices on top, and sprinkle with the salt.

See? Easy!

Beef Balls in Pasta

Ingredients:

For the meatballs

- 6 pounds lean ground beef (supervise the trimming yourself)
- 1/2 cup fresh spinach, chopped
- 1/4 cup red onion, chopped
- 1 tablespoon garlic clove, minced
- 1/2 tablespoon cumin seeds
- Sea salt to taste
- Pepper to taste

For the pasta

- 2 ounces wheat spinach pasta
- 1/8 cup low-sodium marinara
- 2 cups fresh spinach
- 5 cherry tomatoes
- 1 tablespoon low-fat parmesan cheese

Method:

- Preheat the oven to 405 degrees Fahrenheit.
- Place the oil in a pan, and add in the onions.
- Sauté until golden brown.
- In a bowl, add in the minced beef, fresh spinach leaves, sautéed onion, garlic, and various spices.
- Mix them together using your hands, and make small balls out of the mixture.
- Place the balls on a greased baking tray, and place in the oven for 10 to 12 minutes.

- Meanwhile, prepare the sauce by mixing the marinara, spinach, tomatoes, and cheese.
- Cook the pasta until it is al dente.
- Assemble everything on a plate by first placing the pasta, followed by a layer of the sauce, followed by the meatballs, and spoon over the sauce on top.

Chicken Breast Stuffed with Spinach, Tomato, and Feta Cheese, Served with Brown Rice

Ingredients:

- 6 ounces of chicken breast
- ½ cup fresh spinach
- 2 tablespoons feta cheese
- 1 Roma tomato, sliced
- ½ cup brown rice

Method:

- Set the oven to 375 degrees Fahrenheit.
- Cut the chicken breast down the middle so that it spreads out like a butterfly. Make sure that you do not cut all the way through the chicken breast; it should still be attached.
- Season the chicken with your choice of spices and seasonings.
- Spread the chicken breast. On one side, layer the tomato slices, spinach, and feta cheese.
- Fold the chicken breast up like a sandwich, using toothpicks to hold it closed.
- Back the chicken for 18 to 20 minutes or until the chicken is completely cooked.
- While the chicken is cooking, prepare the brown rice. You can add diced onion and garlic for extra flavor if desired.
- Serve the chicken and rice together.

Chickpeas and Lentil Soup

Ingredients:

- 1 can chickpeas, drained
- 1 can black-eyed peas, drained
- 1 cup yellow lentils
- 1 green onion, chopped
- 2 garlic cloves, chopped
- 1 teaspoon olive oil
- 1 green chili, slit
- Salt to taste
- 1 large tomato
- Cilantro to sprinkle

Method:

- Start by placing the chickpeas, beans, and yellow lentils in a large pot of boiling water to which a little salt has been added.
- Once it comes to a boil, cover it and allow the peas and lentils to cook completely.
- Meanwhile, you can sauté the onion and garlic in a little oil and allow them to brown.
- Now add in the chili to the onions and switch off the heat.
- Uncover the peas and stir.
- You can mash them up a bit if you like.
- Add in the onion and garlic, and add 1 cup of water.
- Add in the tomatoes, and cook the soup for around 10 minutes.
- Serve with a sprinkling of cilantro on top.

Chicken Sausage with Peppers

This dish provides a lot of muscle-building power, thanks to the chicken sausage. Plus, it's easy to make and only requires one dish for baking. You can serve it with a salad and some whole grain bread, and you can mix the leftovers with whole grain pasta for a different (but still delicious) second meal.

Ingredients:

- 1 tablespoon olive oil
- 1 pound chicken sausage
- 2 bell peppers, sliced into strips
- 1 red onion, sliced
- 1 teaspoon Worcestershire sauce
- 1 cup marinara sauce
- ¼ cup fresh basil, chopped
- Salt and black pepper to taste

Method:

- Heat the oil in a large skillet over medium heat.
- Add the sausage, and cook until it is browned on all sides.
- Add the pepper and the onions.
- Season with salt and pepper, then cook for 5 minutes.
- Add the Worcestershire sauce and the marinara sauce, and cook for another 5 minutes or until the sausage is thoroughly cooked and the vegetables are tender.
- Garnish the dish with fresh basil and serve.

Baked Fish with Sesame

Ingredients:

- 1 salmon fillet
- 2 tablespoons black sesame seeds
- 1 garlic pod
- 4 to 5 fresh basil leaves
- 1 red onion
- Sea salt to taste
- 2 jalapeño chilies
- 1 tablespoon olive oil
- Fresh cilantro to sprinkle

Method:

- Preheat the oven to 400 degrees Fahrenheit.
- Place the salmon on a greased tray, skin side down.
- Toast the sesame seeds in a pan and allow them to cool.
- Chop the garlic cloves into small pieces and place into the salmon's body.
- Sprinkle the basil leaves all over the fish.
- Sprinkle some of the onion slices on top of the fish, and tuck some under it.
- Sprinkle the jalapeno peppers all over the fish.
- Drizzle some oil on top, followed by the toasted sesame seeds.
- Place the tray in the oven, and bake for 15 to 20 minutes or until fish is fully cooked.
- Serve hot with a sprinkling of fresh cilantro on top.

Sesame and Ginger Tofu with Scallions

This recipe is great for those on a vegetarian or vegan diet, or if you just want to add some variety to your food options. Serve this dish with brown rice for a complete meal.

Ingredients:

- 1 cup extra-firm tofu, diced
- 1 tablespoon extra-virgin olive oil
- ¼ cup scallions, diced
- 2 teaspoons fresh ginger
- 2 tablespoons sesame seeds
- 1 teaspoon smoked paprika (optional)
- Salt to taste

Method:

- Heat the oil in a small skillet over medium heat.
- Add the ginger and the scallions, and sauté for 1 minute.
- Add the tofu, pressing on it with a fork to crumble it.
- Cook until the tofu starts to turn a golden brown.
- Remove the skillet from the stove, and sprinkle the dish with sesame seeds, paprika, and salt.
- Serve the dish directly from the skillet while it is still nice and warm.

Mushroom Sandwiches

Ingredients:

- 5 large Portobello mushrooms, stalks removed
- 2 tablespoons olive oil
- 2 eggs
- 1 avocado
- 2 teaspoons mustard paste
- Salt to taste
- Cayenne pepper to taste
- 2 fresh lettuce leaves

Method:

- Start by smearing the oil over the mushrooms and baking them in a 400-degree Fahrenheit oven for 15 minutes or until they are properly baked
- Meanwhile, boil the eggs, and make sure they are hard boiled.
- Once the mushrooms are done, allow them to cool.
- Cut the eggs in half, and scoop out the yolk.
- Scoop out the avocado flesh, and mix it with the yolk.
- Sprinkle the salt and pepper, and give it a good mix.
- Add the mustard, and mix until well combined.
- Place the mixture in the center of the egg whites.
- Now take one-half of the Portobello and place it upright.
- Place one lettuce leaf over it and one egg half.
- Place another leaf on top, and then cover with another Portobello.
- Serve hot.

Body Cleansing Smoothie

Ingredients:

- 1 scoop protein powder of your choice
- 1 cup chopped kale
- 1 small avocado
- 1 small banana
- 1/4 cup pineapple
- ¼ celery stalk
- 3 strawberries
- Small bundle of wheatgrass
- ¼ cup cooked oatmeal
- 1/4 cup water
- Ice for desired thickness

Method:

- Place the chopped kale, avocado, banana, and pineapple in the blender, and make a smooth paste.
- Add in the protein powder, celery, and wheatgrass and then whizz.
- Now add the oatmeal, water, and ice, and continue to blend.
- The idea is for the flavors to separate and not become one big mess.
- Place in the refrigerator and serve in place of a meal.

Peanut Butter Granola Bites

If you thought that you were going to have to avoid dessert from now on, think again! There are plenty of dessert options out there; you just have to look for ones that will give you beneficial nutritional content while still tasting delicious!

This recipe provides a variety of nutritional benefits: carbs, protein, and omega-3 fats. At only 100 calories per piece, you can eat a piece or two with some fruit for a perfect mid-morning or mid-afternoon snack.

Ingredients:

- 1 cup instant oats
- 1/3 cup natural, creamy peanut butter
- 1/3 cup honey
- 1 tablespoon chia seeds

Method:

- Mix all of the ingredients together, making sure that they are thoroughly combined.
- Refrigerate the mixture for about 30 minutes.
- Once cooled, form balls of about 1 tablespoon each from the mixture, rolling each piece between your fingertips to shape it.
- Store the leftovers in the refrigerator.

Chapter 13: Best Natural Supplements For Lean Muscle Building

It is obvious that we do not get all the needed nutrition through food alone, and so we need to consume supplements in order to supplement our dietary intake.

Let us look at some of the best natural supplements to consume on a daily basis to attain a fit and slim body. These spices and herbs will help you maintain your body weight or lose weight and build muscle by shrinking fat tissue, improving your metabolism, and suppressing your appetite. In addition to these benefits, some of these herbs and spices are sources of antioxidants and could also help to fight heart disease, premature aging, and other chronic diseases.

Remember to always research any product that you are buying, and review the nutritional label if one is provided. Organizations such as the Food and Drug Administration, the Natural Products Association, and the Office of Dietary Supplements will have information about the different products available as well. Always follow the dosage recommendations; more is not necessarily better and can, in fact, be dangerous. Do not hesitate to consult your doctor before introducing any of these supplements into your diet.

Cayenne Pepper

Capsaicin is a chemical found in cayenne pepper that helps in cutting down on fat. It is possible for you to consume a little pepper every day and cut down on the amount of fat present in your body. Cayenne is native to Asia and is extensively used in their cuisine. All you have to do is sprinkle a teaspoonful on your daily meals, and the pepper will do its job, but don't use it in excess as it can burn your throat, and if that happens, then it is best to consume some milk.

Ginger

Ginger is a spice plant that is also native to Asian countries. The plant is fully edible, but the root is dried and used to flavor foods. Ginger is said to help correct ailments of the stomach and encourages the body to dispose of fat instead of storing it. You can chop a little ginger, and add it to your salads or curries or to your smoothies. The idea is to draw from the root's chemical, which helps in transporting fat outside the body. Remember that it is an acquired taste, and you can add a little ginger powder to your tea to reap its benefits.

Cumin

Cumin seeds are also native to Asian cuisine. The seeds have been used in ancient India since time immemorial. They are used for relief from flatulence and for help in eliminating indigestion. Adding a little toasted cumin to your food helps in digesting it better. You will also feel less heavy. You can add it to foods that you think might be fatty. You will end up eating only a little as the cumin seeds will promote a feeling of fullness. Just chewing on a teaspoonful of seeds after dinner can help you lose excess weight and promote digestion.

Cardamom

Cardamom is a spice known for its fragrant aroma and sweet taste. The spice is mainly grown in Asia and is used to flavor sweets and savories alike. All you have to do is acquire some seeds, pound them, and add them to your food. You can also chew on the seeds once you are done eating. The seeds, membrane, and outer skin are all edible and provide the body with ample fiber. You can add some into your daily tea to reap its full benefits.

Ginseng

Ginseng is an herb that has been used in ancient Chinese medicine since time immemorial. The herb comprises the root and bulb of the ginseng plant and is known to possess a whole host of benefits. Metabolism is boosted when a person consumes ginseng, and he or she starts to digest consumed food faster. So the body is left with no time to process the fat and store it, such that the person will not become fat. You can purchase ginseng capsules that have concentrated ginseng. It is also available in powder form, and you can mix some with water and consume.

Fo-ti

Similar to Ginseng, Fo-ti is a Chinese plant that will help to boost your stamina and longevity and will encourage the building of muscle. Fo-ti is most easily obtained by shopping at Chinese markets; while it is a bit more difficult to obtain than Ginseng, its benefits make it worth the extra effort.

Isoleucene

Isoleucene is a compound that is found in many different foods, including soy milk, egg whites, lamb, turkey breast, chicken, tuna, and cottage cheese. Isoleucene helps build your body's protein and is essential for building up muscle mass.

Oats

Oats help build muscle and also are very filling, so they help make you feel full more quickly, dampening your appetite. Not all oats or foods made from oats will provide health benefits. Instant oatmeal, for example, does not provide nearly as much nutritional benefit as regular oatmeal. Preparing your own oatmeal from scratch is a great way to get all of the nutritional benefits and ensure that you are not adding any undesired items to your diet.

Coleus Forskohlii

Also known as Indian coleus, this tropical plant native to India has been used for centuries for a variety of health needs, from heart problems to digestive concerns. Recent studies have shown that coleus forskohlii can help reduce body weight, fat accumulation, and appetite, as well as prevent weight gain. Coleus forskohlii has been reported to sometimes cause increased heart rate and lowered blood pressure, so it may be best to consult with your doctor before trying it out.

Sesamin

Sesamin, which is found in sesame seeds, is a type of compound called lignin. Recent studies have shown that ingesting sesamin can improve the fatty-acid oxidation process by promoting enzyme activity in your liver. As discussed in Chapter 1, fatty acids are a great source of energy for your body, so ingesting sesamin will increase the energy available to your body for muscle building. Combining sesamin with omega-3 fatty acids will improve its effects even more.

Cinnamon

Cinnamon helps enhance your metabolism and also assists in blood sugar regulation. It has also been found to significantly decrease blood sugar levels, LDL (bad) cholesterol, triglycerides, and total cholesterol levels, especially in people with Type-II Diabetes. Regulating blood sugar and decreasing cholesterol levels will help your body function at peak efficiency, which will provide you with the energy and health needed to maintain your exercise plan and build your desired lean muscle mass.

Black Pepper

Black pepper is useful because it contains piperine, a substance that blocks the formation of new fat cells. When black pepper is combined with capsaicin, it has been found to burn as many calories as you would from taking a 20-minute walk. Black pepper has the added benefit of improving the bioavailability of other foods so that your body is able to access as much nutritional value as possible from the foods that you are eating.

Green Tea

The effects of green tea on the body are well known. It is no secret that green tea helps in reducing the free radicals in the body and promotes the growth of healthy cells. Moreover, green tea also helps in reducing body weight and aids in maintaining a slim and trim figure. It is possible for you to lose quite a substantial amount of weight by drinking green tea regularly. You can also consume green tea supplements which will only increase the benefit that your body receives from the herb.

Guarana

Guarana is a tropical fruit with extracts that are said to help build lean muscles in the body. It is an appetite suppressant that curbs hunger pangs, which aids in reducing stress eating. It is used in combination with turmeric to aid in digestion, and it improves the rate of metabolism. You can take it in tablet or capsule form and consume it on a regular basis.

Nettle Leaves

Nettle leaves are loaded with antioxidants and other beneficial nutrients that help build a strong mind and body. It contains Vitamins C and K, which help promote good health. The leaves aid in cleansing the blood and also assist in burning fat.

Turmeric

Turmeric is a spice that is heavily used in Asian cuisine because of its high medicinal value. Curcumin is the chemical present in turmeric and is known to burn fat. You can add a little to your curries or sprinkle a little on your salads. You can also add it to your soup or to your bread dough, and knead it in. Turmeric is also an antiseptic that will strengthen your immunity by a few folds. If you suffer from any internal injuries while performing any of the exercises, then turmeric will help by healing you from the inside.

Dandelion

Dandelion flowers are great for the body. The flower, plant, and leaves are all full of many nutrients, and they are all edible. Dandelion aids in digestion and helps in digesting even the toughest of fats. It is used by several celebrities to lose weight and remain slim for long. It is loaded with beta-carotene and Vitamin K1, which help bring the blood sugar levels down and control insulin levels in the body. You can consume dandelion tea and also chop and add the stalks and leaves to your salads.

Mustard Seeds

Mustard is extremely beneficial in fighting off fat in the body. Mustard seeds are said to boost the body's metabolism by 25%, and in fact, it is probably by the highest margin. It is possible for you to improve your digestion just by consuming a teaspoon of mustard paste or adding 2 tablespoons of the seeds to your curries. According to recent studies, consuming a little will help you burn 45 calories of fat an hour.

Nicholas Bjorn

Chapter 14: What To Avoid – Food Edition

So far, we have been dealing with what is healthy for you, your body, and your fitness and nutrition plans. However, this chapter with deal with the opposites or what is unhealthy and bad for you and your body and what can nullify all the effort you have been putting into healthy living.

Among the things that are proven unhealthy or even devastating in the long term, food is the first that comes to mind. Unhealthy food includes sugary drinks, pizzas, white bread, margarine, vegetable oils, pastries, cookies and cakes, French fries, ice cream, candy bars, processed meat, cheese, artificial sweeteners, and many others.

Sugary Drinks

If we were on a mission to find the unhealthiest product today, we would definitely end up with added sugar. However, it must be emphasized that not all sources of sugar are bad. In the sea of unhealthy products full of sugar, the most important or the unhealthiest are sugary drinks. Many people don't actually realize that drinks also have calories, and because of that, they fail to understand that drinks can also be bad for health. Sugary drinks include sodas, fruit punches, lemonades, energy drinks, and other drinks with added sugar. Constant consumption of sugary drinks leads to obesity, which can have devastating effects on the human body. Surprisingly, fruit juices are also included in this category. Although they have more nutrients, they also contain very high levels of sugar and calories, which can be very easily neglected by people.

In order to avoid what was previously mentioned, people must totally abandon the practice of consuming sugary drinks and search for alternatives, such as water, soda water, tea, and many others. Among the drinks with the most sugar per ounce are the fruit juices with a range of 4.75 to 7.15 grams of sugar per ounce, followed by regular sodas, energy drinks, ice tea/coffee, and sports drinks.

While you may think that drinks with artificial sweeteners would be a great alternative to sugary drinks, artificial sweeteners can actually be just as harmful. In fact, artificial sweeteners have been shown to increase one's appetite for sweet food. While the cause of this has not been confirmed, it is likely due to the body increasing insulin secretion when sweeteners are eaten in anticipation of the glucose that will appear in the blood. When the glucose does not come because the sweetener is artificial, your blood sugar will drop, and you will experience increased hunger.

Pizzas

Pizza is the ultimate favorite food of so many of us. However, only a few of us understand the danger that pizza poses on our health. Similar to sugary drinks, pizza is also one of the reasons for the growing rate of obesity in the world. As regards the number of calories, 100 grams of pizza contain 266 calories, which is for sure a number you don't want to be a part of your daily eating habits. Aside from calories, some pizzas contain 1,620 mg of sodium and 33 grams of fat. One slice of cheese pizza also contains 5 grams of sugar. However, not all pizzas are marked as unhealthy. In order to avoid the high intake of calories, fat, sugar, and other unhealthy nutrients, people often choose a vegetable pizza. Vegetable pizza contains Vitamins A and C and more fiber in comparison to cheese or meat pizza. Add to this some veggie toppings, such as mushrooms, spinach, tomatoes, or onions, and you will get not only an amazing pizza but also a healthy intake of vitamins and other healthy nutrients.

White Bread

In the majority of cases, white bread is made of wheat, which contains gluten, and because of this, white bread is not good for people who are sensitive to gluten. However, white bread is not bad only for gluten-sensitive people but also for everybody else. White bread is mostly made of refined wheat, the healthy nutrients of which are reduced to a minimum because of the refining process. What you get in the end are pure calories, which can result in high blood pressure for some people. If you want to use bread, it is better to use whole grain bread instead of white bread. Whole grain bread contains a lot more vitamins, minerals, and fiber than white bread. All of this provides you with more energy throughout the day. One slice of white bread has 66 calories, 0.82 grams of fat, 12.65 grams of carbs, and 1.91 grams of protein. Yes, you do get some protein with white bread, but the damage the white bread is causing is much bigger than the benefits of the proteins it contains.

Margarine

Can you imagine a time when margarine was considered to be healthier than butter? Well, that was the case until recently, when it was proven that margarine is much more dangerous for your health than butter. There is a debate about whether butter is good for your health on not, but it is definitely healthier than the margarine, and the reason for this is that butter is made up of natural ingredients while margarine, on the other hand, is made of artificial ingredients in order to look and taste just like the butter. Some margarine contains trans fats that, just like saturated fat, elevate blood pressure and have negative effects on your health. There are several types of margarine: stick margarine, light margarine, margarine with phytosterols, and several others. Only one teaspoon of stick margarine already has between 80 and 100 calories, between 9 and 11 grams of fat, and 2 grams of saturated fat. Butter or margarine it is not really important because there is no big difference in their effects on your body. Both are unhealthy and may cause some serious problems.

Pastries, Cookies, and Cakes

The majority of products from this category are proven unhealthy. Often, pastries are made of refined sugar, butter, refined flour, and added fats. The combination of all of these can cause serious problems for the human body. The biggest danger that can be caused by such products is diabetes. All pastries, cookies, cakes, ice cream, and other desserts contain a large number of calories, and if you are not able to burn those calories at the gym or through some other exercise, they will be stored in your body as body fat. However, just like every other unhealthy food, there is a healthy counterpart for desserts. Some desserts provide you with healthy nutrients. Those healthy nutrients can be found in fruits. So if you want to have dessert, try and find one that does not contain a large amount of sugar, fat, or butter. Your body will thank you for it.

Instant Ramen

Wait, what? Instant ramen is bad? But that's all I've been eating in college! No, but seriously, instant ramen is definitely not healthy. If you think about it for a second, instant ramen has a ridiculous amount of salt in it. It can have up to 2,000 mg of salt, which is definitely not healthy for your body. On average, your daily intake should not exceed 1,500 mg of sodium. Most people already eat some foods with sodium before dinner time. Having instant ramen to help you get through finals week or just as a quick meal is the last thing you should be doing. If you regularly eat instant ramen and then cut it out of your diet, you'll notice a lot of differences in your body, including not being as thirsty and feeling better overall. Sodium is okay, just in moderation.

French Fries And Potato Chips

One of the unhealthiest foods out there is definitely French fries. Potatoes, in general, are healthy, but potatoes in French fries are everything but healthy. Several studies conducted recently in different parts of the world identify French fries as one of the reasons why people are gaining more and more weight and, due to that, are becoming more and more unhealthy. One of the reasons why fries are unhealthy is because they contain bad fats, and by now, we all know what kind of danger bad fats are for our health. The second reason why fries are considered unhealthy is because they are made of bad carbohydrates. In the body, potato converts to sugar, and if we are not able to spend that sugar through exercise, it remains in the body in the form of fat. Another reason why we consider fries unhealthy is because they contain trans fats, which are dangerous when in relation to heart diseases. Also, these trans fats are linked to diabetes and certain types of cancer. In the process of making French fries, all good or healthy elements are removed from the potato, and what is left are only the unhealthy elements that have no nutritional value. As regards the number of calories, a medium portion of French fries has 365 calories and 17 grams of fat.

Much of the information above also applies to potato chips, unfortunately. While potato chips are a favorite snack for many, they are very high in calories and provide virtually no nutritional benefit. In addition, potato chips tend to come in servings that make it far too easy to eat way more than you should.

Instead of potato chips, you can eat plain popped corn, whole grain crackers, or cut-up vegetables.

Alcohol

You may not want to hear it, but alcohol is one of the first things that should be eliminated (or at least greatly reduced) from your diet if you are trying to lose weight and build muscle. Like potato chips above, alcohol provides very little, if any, nutritional value – it is essentially empty calories. As with potato chips, it is hard to regulate the amount that you are taking in; drinking some alcohol tends to lead to drinking more alcohol. The type of alcohol is important: beer is definitely associated with weight gain, whereas wine (in moderation) can be beneficial.

Ice Cream

While ice cream does have some nutritional value, unlike many of the food items discussed in this chapter, it is still very unhealthy. Ice cream is very high in calories and is usually full of sugar. As with the other foods on this list, it is also difficult to eat just a little ice cream, and it usually comes in servings that make it hard to limit your intake. If you absolutely need to have ice cream every once in a while, try making your own; you can use less sugar and healthier ingredients, like fresh fruit and yogurt.

Specialty Coffee Drinks

Fancy coffee drinks with a variety of delicious flavorings are a popular option for many people, but unfortunately, these drinks tend to be extremely high in calories. The problems with these coffee drinks are the same as those with sugary drinks discussed above: empty calories and little, if any, nutritional value. Moreover, we tend to add sugar (or artificial sweeteners) and milk or cream to these drinks, increasing the caloric content even further.

Plain, black coffee can actually help with weight loss because caffeine will boost your metabolism. Adding low-fat or part-skim milk is fine, but try to avoid adding sugar or sweeteners.

Candy Bars

Eating candy regularly can have negative effects on your health. Eating too many candies can result in the body having too much sugar and fats. Candy bars and candies, in general, are full of sugar, and we have already seen what kind of consequences too much sugar intake can have on your body and on your health. Aside from sugar, candies contain a large number of calories. Some candies may contain between 250 and 280 calories per portion. For example, a Snickers candy bar has 280 calories, 14 grams of fat, and 30 grams of sugar; a Twix candy bar has 250 calories and 12 grams of fat; and a Mars candy bar has 230 calories and 8.6 grams of fat. Consequently, eating too much candy every day will result in too many calories in your body which would have devastating effects on your health. Of course, it is impossible to abandon candies, just like any other food previously mentioned, for good, but it is necessary to have control over the intake of the aforementioned food. Otherwise, the consequences to your health may be devastating.

Any Foods High In Added Sugar

While this applies to most of the foods discussed above, sugar is added to many foods, and some of these may surprise you. This can include breakfast cereals, low-fat products, and granola bars. In fact, low-fat and fat-free foods are often supplemented with additional sugar to make up for the flavor lost from removing the fat content.

Other food products that likely contain much higher amounts of sugar than you would expect include commercial salad dressings (make your own for a healthy alternative), whole wheat products (look for whole grain instead), sports drinks, and foods advertised as "low-carb." You should also keep in mind that just because food is labeled as organic, vegan, or gluten-free does not automatically mean that it is healthy: many of these foods are processed and contain high levels of sugar.

The bottom line is that you should always look at the nutritional label before picking food in order to avoid surprises, such as higher than expected sugar content.

Processed Meat

Unlike unprocessed meat, processed meat is proven to have negative effects on your health. Several studies around the world indicated that some serious diseases, such as colon cancer, diabetes, and heart diseases, could all be the result of the consumption of the processed meat. If we were to look for a definition of processed meat, it would state that processed meat refers to meat that has been cured, salted, dried, canned, and smoked. In the category of processed meat, we can include hot dogs, sausages, salami, bacon, and ham. According to some studies, processed meat contains N-nitroso compounds that are proven to be cancer-causing elements. The most important thing about the intake of processed meat is self-control. You must be able to determine the maximum amount of processed meat you are going to eat, and decide on what type of processed meat you will be eating because not all types of processed meat are equally unhealthy.

As we have seen from this chapter, it is hard to live or, in this case, to eat healthy because all of our favorite foods seem to be the most dangerous ones. All of the food previously mentioned in this chapter bears a level of danger that can have serious consequences in the future. Limited consumption of the mentioned food doesn't necessarily have bad effects on your health, but the constant, everyday consumption of such food has been proven to be devastating. Sometimes, it is important to have a "cheat day" – a day where you will eat this kind of food, but the consumption of such food needs to be limited to as little as possible.

Chapter 15: What To Avoid – Exercise Edition

Just like not all food is healthy, not all exercises are beneficial for your body and your health. In order to get perfect muscles, we often neglect the advice of influential people who are constantly warning us about the dangers of certain exercises in the gym and outside.

The following chapter provides a list of several exercises that were marked by experts as dangerous because of poor performance or negative effects that they have on the human body.

Bench Dips

While doing this exercise, your arms are by your side, and your palms are facing forward. The problem with this exercise is that your shoulders become more vulnerable to injury the further you move from your position. Some consequences of this exercise include abrasions to the deltoid, cuff muscles, and bursae.

If the goal of this exercise is to train our triceps, then there is a better exercise than doing bench dips. Instead, you could use parallel bars where your hands are parallel to each other, and your head leans behind where it belongs.

Chin-Ups And Pull-Ups

The problem with this exercise is that many people try to do chin-ups before they are physically and mentally ready for such an exercise. In such cases, doing this exercise results in injuries that prevent you from doing any other workout.

An even more dangerous exercise would be pull-ups. The difference between chin-ups and pull-ups is that pull-ups don't involve lifting the body up with your hands but rather lifting the body up with the help of your hips. This exercise became popular with the introduction of CrossFit. CrossFit, being a high-intensity combination of several exercise interval training is not for everybody. CrossFit requires extreme physical readiness. Consequently, every exercise from CrossFit can be dangerous for people who are not physically ready for such a regimen.

Deadlifts

Deadlifts are very demanding and technically complex for the entire body, and they are often done incorrectly. The biggest danger coming from this exercise concerns the spine. It is possible for you to damage your disks if you do deadlifts in the wrong manner, and damage to the spine is always devastating. One of the most common mistakes when doing deadlifts is the fact that people often lift weights using their backs or only their hands without using the core and the entire body. Just like all other exercises, physical readiness is crucial for this exercise. A lack of physical readiness often results in back, hand, or muscle injury.

Wide-Grip Lat Pulldown

This exercise is used to train the muscles of your back. Although a lot of people would say that this exercise was very useful for them, they would neglect to mention the problems that occurred during or after that exercise. The biggest risk with this exercise lies in the consequences that it can have on your shoulders.

In order to perform this exercise, you must rotate your shoulders as much as you can so that you are able to pull down the lat behind your neck. Here again, the muscles of your shoulders are exposed the most, and this can result in neck strain or strain on the top of your shoulders.

Once again, adequate preparation is crucial if you want to perform this exercise successfully. However, as is the case with many of the previously mentioned exercises, there is a replacement exercise that you can do instead of a wide-grip lat pulldown and reduce the risk of injury, and that exercise is the front pulldown.

The Seated Rotation Machine

The seated rotation machine is an exercise that works your hips and abs while sitting. This exercise is proven to be very stressful to your lower back because all emphasis is on the lower back, and a sitting position is not something suitable for doing exercises. When doing this exercise, your body sits while you twist your hips or torso from one side to another, which results in significant pressure on your lower back.

Instead of putting such pressure on your lower back by doing such an exercise, you could do a standing twist of your torso that, unlike seated twisting, would not put so much pressure on your lower back.

Upright Rows

The problem with this exercise is that it places a lot of strain on the shoulder joint, which exposes the shoulder and upper arm to injury. If you are going to do this exercise, try initiating the lift by driving with your legs and turning it into a high pull movement instead of a rowing movement. This will allow you to move the weight differently, thus placing less strain on your shoulder joint.

Curtsy Lunges

This type of lunge is different from the traditional lunge in that your knee travels across the body in front rather than forward and backward. While it provides a great burn for your thigh muscles, the movement involved in this exercise violates the basic principle that your knee, hip, and shoulder joints should be kept in alignment when you are doing load-bearing exercises. This exercise introduces stress to the hip socket, as well as the iliotibial (IT) band and tensor fasciae latae (TFL) muscle in your knee.

Stick to traditional lunges instead. If you want to make it more challenging, you can add a height differential: stand on a low platform and lunge forward or backward off of the platform.

Ab Machines

While this is a machine rather than a specific exercise, it is still a good idea to avoid it. The problem with ab machines is that they encourage poor posture and can cause muscle imbalances because they tend to target only one or two muscles in your core when there are many different muscles in that area that need to be targeted for a proper, balanced workout.

Anything That Causes Actual Pain

Yes, working out can be uncomfortable, and it can (and should) cause your muscles to ache or burn – that means that you are using your muscles and building your strength. But anytime that you feel actual pain – sharp and sudden – you should stop immediately. Either you are pushing your body past its limits, or you are doing something that your body is not meant to do, and both of those should be avoided if you do not want to injure yourself.

As we have seen in this chapter, not all exercises are good for your body and your health. Several of them actually seem to have more negative than positive effects. The most crucial thing to know before going for a workout is your physical readiness. It is crucial to know whether your body is ready for such training and to understand the limits of your own body. Doing exercises that your body can't handle is a path that leads towards imminent injury. No amount of pull-ups or twisting can compensate for a permanent back or muscle injury.

Remember, just because you see people doing it on TV does not mean that you and everybody else can do the same exercises. People who are very experienced and have a high level of fitness will be able to do certain exercises and movements properly, whereas a beginner will likely injure him or herself. Try and stick to the exercises that were discussed in earlier chapters of this book, or work with a professional trainer – at least at the start – to make sure that you are doing your exercises properly and that you are not pushing your body further than is healthy. You can work your way up to more difficult and challenging exercises, but if you injure yourself by doing too much too soon, then you are not going to achieve your fitness goals.

Chapter 16: The Importance Of Cardio Training

Although some people hate the words "cardio training," they are bound to witness the benefits that come after some time. On the other hand, for some people, cardio training has become something that they cannot get enough of. Cardio or cardiovascular exercise can be described as any type of movement that results in an elevated heart rate and increased blood circulation throughout the body.

Cardio training or cardiovascular exercises are mostly performed in order to burn off calories because they are proven to be among the most efficient ways to lose weight. However, cardio training alone does not help in losing weight. The crucial point here is the ratio of calories burned to those taken in. If the number of calories burned by cardio training is greater than the number consumed, you will lose weight.

Aside from the benefits of losing weight, cardio training also helps increase endurance, contributes to a better mental state and healthy skin, increases blood flow, lowers heart rate when resting, and improves metabolism. Thus, the benefits of cardio training are not only reflected in the body but also in the mind. An increase in cardio also means you are more likely to have more energy and sleep better at night. This can really help you feel better every morning, knowing that you have enough energy to get through the day.

There are several ways in which cardio training can be done, and they include: running or jogging, brisk walking, cycling, swimming, aerobic dance, cross-country skiing, and many others.

Running Or Jogging

According to some studies, regular exercise that includes 150 minutes (30 minutes per day, five days a week) has a great amount of health benefits that cannot be compared to any doctor's prescription. Running has also been proven to help in the prevention of diabetes, heart diseases, high blood pressure, obesity, and a number of other health issues. Running, just like the majority of other exercises, helps in overcoming hard times or depression periods, as well as in coping with anxiety and stress. One of the clearer effects of running is losing weight for sure. Running is proven to be one of the fastest ways to burn calories. Running can also play an important role in strengthening your knees, and it can have a positive effect on other bones as well. Some even claim that running helps in the prevention of certain cancers, and it prolongs the life span of people. Aside from all of this, running out in the open provides you with the opportunity to enjoy the fresh air instead of being in a closed space.

Runners seem to be happier than those who do not run, so if you want a happier and more fulfilling life, take up running and enjoy the benefits that come with it so you could enjoy life in full. For 30 minutes a day, your life can change in ways you never thought were possible. All the previously mentioned benefits of running can be applied to jogging as well. Just like running, jogging helps you in increasing your muscle mass without having to do any heavy lifting. The reduction of the risk for osteoporosis is also linked to these two physical activities.

If running outside just isn't an option, you can go to a gym and get on a treadmill. While you won't get the same outside air that you would otherwise, you can still do your workout. Treadmills are great because they can still mimic running up a hill. It almost seems harder just because a treadmill could keep the hill up for an indefinite amount of time, but if you do have the choice to run or jog outside, then you should definitely go for that before looking at getting on a treadmill.

It is important to keep in mind some of the risks that may come with running. People who have bad knees will likely have a harder time running because it is very harsh on your knees. In order to alleviate some of that pain, you need to make sure your quads, hips, and glutes are all strong enough to stop that from happening. Having any of these be weak will only cause issues in your knees.

Another common issue is stomach pain. The constant hitting of your feet on the pavement can be jarring on your stomach. If you are just starting out, you should make sure to eat two to three hours before you go on a run, and try to make it something light. The heavier your breakfast is when you go for a run, the more likely you will either be sick or have diarrhea. None of that is a good thing, especially when you are just starting out. This one bad experience could cause you never to want to run again.

There's one thing many people forget about when they go running for the first few times. Chafing is an annoying thing that can be very painful. It might seem impossible to stop from happening, but it is actually possible to stop it. For this, you'll want to make sure to properly lubricate any areas you think will be rubbed against. You should also make sure to wear underwear made of a wicking material rather than cotton. Cotton will only make the issue worse, no matter how well you lubricate it. If you can afford to spend a little extra money, you should definitely buy some high-quality wicking fabric. It will last longer and work much better than some low-quality materials.

Running and jogging are both great ideas to get your heart pumping. It's something basic that anyone can go out and do. If you properly take care of your body before, during, and after a run, then you'll be able to do this for years to come. There are people who are older who will still get up every day and go for a jog around their neighborhood. That being said, this isn't for everyone, but there are other ways to get your cardio in for the day.

Brisk Walking

Who would have thought that such a simple activity as walking can have such benefits of your health? This is the case with brisk walking. Brisk walking, in essence, is energetic and quick walking that includes heavy breathing. When you find yourself brisk walking and you feel that your heart rate has gone up, then you can be sure that brisk walking is useful for your body. Just like running and jogging, brisk walking enables better blood circulation throughout the body. Brisk walking also enables you to do this activity in pairs or in groups, although conversation while brisk walking will be a little difficult due to the heavy breathing. Just like running and jogging, brisk walking outside, in the park, or in the forest enables you to breathe fresh air and absorb the required Vitamin D.

Walking is a very good option for those who are just starting on their exercise journey because it is easy on the body, requires no special equipment other than a good pair of shoes, and is not at all intimidating. It can also be done inside on the treadmill for days when the weather makes it too unpleasant to exercise outside. While the treadmill may not be as enjoyable as walking outside, it does have the benefit of reducing the impact on your joints, and it allows you to monitor your speed, heart rate, and other important data.

Walking at a speed of 3.0 miles per hour is a good starting point for beginners. Try to work up to at least 4.0 miles per hour eventually to get your heart rate to a level that will promote weight loss. You can also incorporate hills into your walk to increase your heart rate and get more of a muscle workout.

Losing weight is not an easy job. It takes a long time to lose weight depending on the amount you want to lose. Walking is definitely one of the best ways to accomplish such a goal. You don't have to go to the gym or buy expensive equipment. All you have to do to start losing weight is to start walking to work, school, university, and back. Several studies have proven that people who regularly walk, whether to work, school, university, or for leisure for several years, weigh less than people who do not walk very often. One of the benefits of regular walking is better posture, because walking in the right way will create a habit of walking right.

Cycling

Cycling is a sport, or rather, an exercise that is suitable for everybody. Aside from the fact that cycling is an amazing workout in general, in provides a way for losing weight and becoming healthier. There are numerous benefits of cycling, but the most striking or obvious one is weight loss. Aside from weight loss, cycling is a workout for the entire body in general. There is hardly any group of muscles that is not affected by the benefits of cycling. Cycling is a cheap exercise, so there is no burden of spending a lot of money on buying equipment or memberships in local gyms. Moreover, it provides you with the opportunity to enjoy the nature and fresh air, which also contributes benefits to your lungs.

It is important to emphasize that cycling does not require any special training. Given that almost everybody has learned to ride a bike in their childhood, it won't be difficult for anybody to get back on the bike and to start enjoying the ride and losing weight. When you ride a bike, even your heart is going through a workout. When you ride a bike, your heart rate is elevated, and blood flow throughout the body is increased. A bike is also a very good means of transport. Consequently, you can use your bike to go work or perform your daily responsibilities, leave your car at the parking lot, lose weight, and avoid traffic jams at the same time. Cycling in groups also provides you with the opportunity to socialize more and to spend more time with your friends.

Riding a bike is a low-impact workout, which means it won't be super harsh on your body. You'll be able to go for a much longer period of time without having to stop because of discomfort. Moreover, because of the low impact, injuries will occur less often. Of course, this also has to do with how to take care of your body outside of cycling. If you don't properly take care of your body when you are riding your bike, then injuries will happen way more often.

This can also increase your stamina and aerobic fitness. A great thing about cycling is that it can be a simple workout to get your heart working, or you can make it an intense, full body workout. This makes it incredibly beneficial in the long run, as you can mix it up every day, sometimes doing high–intensity workouts and then doing a day of low-impact work.

There are some great benefits that come with cycling. For one, it can improve your cardiovascular health, which can decrease the risk of heart attack and stroke, two things that can be very detrimental to your health. Cycling can be incredibly helpful for your joints, especially as you get older. Joints can become achy and painful to walk on and use. Cycling can increase the mobility of your joints, making them even easier to use and significantly less painful.

What's even better about cycling is you can burn up to 650 calories per hour of moderate biking. This is such a great overall workout and can be incredibly fun. You can explore new places, go on the road, or go through the woods as long as there's a decent path. Cycling can make a huge difference in your life by helping you lose weight, helping with any depression or anxiety that you have, and just making you feel better with your own body.

Swimming

Swimming, or the perfect exercise as it is called on many occasions, is the best way for you to exercise all your muscles, as well as to enhance your cardio performance. Swimming as an exercise helps you improve your muscle definition and increase your strength. Swimming also has a positive effect on bone mass, which was previously doubted, but recent studies have shown the positive effect of swimming on this aspect.

One of the best benefits of the swimming is losing weight. Depending on the type of swimming, it can burn more calories than running. In the beginning of this chapter, we talked about how running is efficient in burning calories, and now, we see that certain types of swimming are even more efficient than running. For example, an hour of freestyle swimming will burn 100 calories, an hour of breaststroke swimming will burn 60 calories, an hour of backstroke swimming will burn 80 calories, and an hour of butterfly swimming will burn 150 calories.

Swimming is also a great way of reducing stress levels and increasing your self-esteem. A healthy body doesn't mean much if the mind is not in the right place. Thus, aside from benefits for the body, swimming also provides exercise for the mind. Just like many other activity from this chapter, swimming also reduces the risk of certain diseases, especially heart disease. It is interesting to note that when athletes suffer an injury, their road to recovery leads them to the pool, where they can heal their injuries by swimming. This indicates that swimming can have healing benefits as well.

Swimming is a great exercise for people of any age. It's not a super high-intensity workout, unless you want it to be. If you wanted to, you could easily do a ten-minute workout in the pool and then play something like water polo. It would be a very intense workout, as you burn a lot of calories playing water polo. Someone around 130 pounds can burn up to 590 calories for every hour of play, and someone around 180 pounds can burn 817 calories. This means you should definitely eat a good meal a few hours before getting into the pool or you might get sick from not eating.

Outside of that, there are so many different types of swimming you can do. There's freestyle swimming, breaststroke, backstroke, sidestroke, the butterfly, and the elementary backstroke. There's also the doggy paddle, but that's more of a thing kids might do. Even that can make you burn 400 calories per hour, if you did have the desire to do that.

How fast you go and how long you do the stroke will really put into perspective the amount of working out you just did. For every hour you spend on a specific stroke, you'll burn more calories. If you go even faster, you'll add to the calories that you've burned. You'll even burn more calories if you just goof off in the pool. The more serious you take something, the more calories you'll be able to burn because you're pushing your body to do more than it's probably used to doing.

If you don't want to focus so much on specific strokes, you still get a big workout from swimming. Maybe it's the middle of the summer, and you want to go to the beach with your family. If you have kids, you'll probably be running around the beach, chasing your younger kids or making sandcastles. Then, you'll go into the water and swim, either by yourself or with your family. Any time spent in the water is a good workout. If you spend one day at the beach, you might be able to burn a thousand calories or more. Of course, if your ideal day at the beach is sitting in the sun and tanning, then you probably won't be burning a whole lot of calories.

Swimming is easily the best kind of exercise to do if you want a whole body workout. Every part of your body is engaged when you go to the pool or the beach and start swimming. Even after you get out of the pool, you'll still be burning some calories from the workout you just did, making it very beneficial long after your workout, not to mention that swimming is also a lot of fun to do. There aren't many exercises that can be considered fun right from the beginning, but this is easily one of them.

Aerobic Dance

Aerobic dance, or aerobic exercise, is pretty much any activity that results in sweat, heavy breathing, and elevated heart beat rate as compared with when you are in a resting position. The aim of this kind of exercises is to strengthen your heart and lungs, as well as to train your body to be able to deliver oxygen more quickly and in a more efficient way.

There are several benefits that your body will thank you after you take on aerobic exercises. Aerobic exercises enhance the amount of oxygen that the cardiovascular system uses. With this kind of exercise, your body increases its endurance, and you are able to prolong your training time. It also helps in reducing the level of stress, anxiety, or depression. Given that you feel pretty tired after the workout, you will sleep better after the training. Most importantly, aerobic dance or exercise is a fun and very effective way of losing weight.

One of the best and the most interesting ways of aerobic dances is **Zumba**. This type of dance is a combination of Latin, International, and Salsa music, and it makes you move to the rhythm of the music. Zumba is a great full body dance workout that tones your entire body. Given that the dances are fun, you'll likely come back to them over and over again, so they won't easily lose their excitement, and coming back will help you lose weight. Moreover, it gives pretty good results. People are able to lose a significant amount of weight within a few months. That being said, you should definitely eat well while you are exercising if you want the best results.

Stress is something everyone has, but Zumba might be able to make your life a little less stressful. There is a lot you can do in Zumba that takes your mind away from whatever is bothering you. Along with reducing stress, it can also reduce symptoms of depression and anxiety. This aerobic dance is accessible to a lot of people of every age, so you can get other people to do the workout with you, making it even more fun. Plus, finding classes is super easy. There are Zumba classes in almost every city, if you want to take part in the workout with a group of people. Alternatively, you can buy a DVD from a store or online and do these workouts at home. There are plenty of beginner workouts for you to try.

Jazzercise is another type of aerobic dance. These sessions last for 60 minutes, and they will make you sweat, get your heart rate up, and help reduce the signs of heart diseases. It is a unique blend of aerobics, yoga, Pilates, kickboxing, and resistance training. This easily makes it a whole body workout and one that might be a little tough to get into as a beginner. This doesn't mean that it's restricted to one group of people. Anyone can go to a class and try this out. It is a great workout that will burn tons of calories – up to 600 an hour. Jazzercise became wildly popular in the 1970s and still has plenty of classes all over the world, so you can definitely find one near you.

Belly dancing is also a very interesting and very useful type of aerobic dance. It comes from the Arabic countries, and your torso is the most used area of your body in this exercise. This exercise is pretty tough and can be incredibly rewarding. There is a lot of work that goes into this exercise. You might not believe it, but you can be any weight when you go into belly dancing. There's no rule that states you need to be under a certain weight in order to belly dance. In fact, belly dancing is simply moving your body in ways that it can be moved. There aren't any crazy movements that your body wouldn't be able to do under normal circumstances.

It might be a bit of a shock to your body when you first start, but after some practice, you'll find it a lot easier to belly dance. You'll also start seeing some results. You can burn anywhere from 250 to 300 calories an hour if you continuously work. Some classes will be more intense than others. You might be in one class that has you always keeping your heart rate up and then go to another class where it's much more slow-paced. You'll be working on specific things rather than just keeping your heart rate up. All of this depends on what you want out of this exercise and how fast you want to move.

Ballroom dancing is probably not something you would expect to be an aerobic dance, but it still is in that field. It's a low-intensity dance, so there won't be a ton of quick weight loss, but with a lot of practice and working on it, you can still lose some weight. Obviously, ballroom dancing means you are paired up with another person, so you'll need to have a partner in order to do these dances. There are many types of dancing involved in ballroom, including the waltz, tango, salsa, Vietnamese waltz, and quickstep.

The tango and the salsa in particular are a little more of a workout than, say, the waltz will be. They require a lot of quick dance moves with your partner, which means faster footwork and faster reflexes. Overall, ballroom dancing can really tone your muscles. This is a great one to do after you've already begun the weight loss process, as you'll be able to tone your body as you lose weight. As an added bonus, ballroom dancing has been proven to help keep your bones strong. You can actually burn anywhere from 200 to 400 calories per hour of ballroom dancing, depending on the intensity.

Just like all other exercises, it is crucially important to pre-warm up before taking up any kind of these aerobic dances. Moreover, with these different types of aerobic dance, you will have a boost of energy after you start doing these exercises daily or every few days. Your body will be used to working out, so you'll be more tired at night, making it easier for you to fall asleep.

Cross-country Skiing

One of the most surprising activities on this list is cross-country skiing. It is pretty much a limited-access activity, but those who have the opportunity to try cross-country skiing emphasize the importance and benefits of such a workout. Cross-country skiing is an activity that completely relies on your ability and the strength of your body, and because of that, cross-country skiing is considered to be one of the most beneficial workouts currently.

Cross-country skiing burns a lot of calories because it combines the lower and upper body workout while your muscles are constantly being pulled and pushed. Cross-country skiing burns up to 1,122 calories for one hour of the activity, which is a really staggering number. No other activity burns so many calories per hour. In comparison, an hour of competitive boxing burns 816 calories per hour, a stair-stepper burns 612 calories per hour, and football burns 612 calories per hour. Just like many other exercises, cross-country skiing helps increase your resistance and endurance and provides you with a great level of physical fitness.

Fresh winter air, which is full of clean air, does wonders to your lungs and heart by increasing the level of oxygen produced by the cardiovascular system in your body. It is also a great opportunity to spend time outdoors while enjoying the scenery and having a good time with your friends.

This is a full body workout for sure. So many parts of your body are used as you go along, even if you don't feel it at the time. It's pretty interesting when you go cross-country skiing and then realize later that you're really sore. Some of that has to do with the cold air making it hard to tell, but it doesn't really feel like all that much work.

Believe it or not, cross-country skiing is considered a low-impact workout. When you think about it, all you're doing is skiing on a relatively flat surface. There aren't any heavy weights to lift or hard impact on your knees. There might be some gentle hills, but that's all.

Have you ever heard of runner's high? This is when a bunch of endorphins are released into your body and generally give you a big jump in energy. They also make you really focus on what you're currently doing, which then, in turn, makes that task easier to do. This is something many people experience when doing cross-country skiing. It gives them the extra push they might need to get through a long session out on the snow.

Snowshoeing is another big calorie burner. You can burn over 1,000 calories per hour doing this as well. Plus, snowshoeing actually has even more benefits, with the added bonus of being a mix of strength, agility, balance, and endurance. This is a lot slower paced than cross-country skiing, but it's also a huge workout. This is a low-impact form of exercise that is safe for many people to do. Even though you're essentially walking, it can burn way more calories than just simple walking can.

You can vary how intense your workout is by what type of snow you walk on. Powdery snow on a hill will be a lot harder and more intense than walking on flat terrain. This is a great workout for people who usually do it. The main reason why you burn so many more calories is the mix of using different muscle groups and the cold that you're walking in. This combination makes it a lot easier to burn calories and shed off weight.

Both of these winter exercises are incredible for your body. They work the body in ways you might not have thought possible, but there are some great results that come from that. Even if you usually do workouts inside, it's always great to go out into the cold and do some super effective workouts.

Jumping Rope

While jumping rope may seem like more of a childhood activity than an actual exercise, it actually provides a great workout and is a fantastic way to get your heart rate up and warm up for your workout. Jumping rope is not going to be an entire workout in itself because very few people would be able to jump for longer than 10 or 15 minutes at most. For the best results, mix it in with another exercise, as it's very difficult to keep that going for a long period of time. What it does do is burn a lot of calories in a short time and get your heart pumping so that your body moves quickly into fat-burning status, thereby allowing you to get the most out of the rest of your workout. Jumping rope also has the benefit of being cheap, given that you can find a jumping rope for a few dollars at your local toy store.

Jumping rope is a high-impact workout, but it is actually less impactful on the body than running is, as long as it's done properly. It strengthens both the upper and lower body, along with giving some awesome cardio, especially when done quickly. This is also great to do in order to see how your body works and just becoming more aware of your body in every way. Jumping rope is something that can be done with some friends or even kids.

Kickboxing

Kickboxing is an intense workout, burning up to 750 calories per hour. It has also been reported to be a highly effective stress-reliever and provides some self-defense training. If you are intimidated by kickboxing classes and doing this type of workout in front of others, you can get started at home by buying a kickboxing video. If you do better with exercise that combines with socialization, then join a kickboxing class. Many fitness companies offer these classes, but there are also specialized gyms that provide kickboxing and similar courses. Whichever option you choose, make sure that it is one that will motivate you to actually do the exercise.

Kickboxing combines martial arts, boxing, and aerobics. It can also help improve balance, coordination, flexibility, and self-confidence, all while teaching you some basic self-defense. You have to admit, kickboxing looks pretty appealing, especially to those who are a little younger. Kickboxing can be pretty demanding, so those who are very overweight, have physical limitations, or are significantly out of shape might want to look at something else first. Then from that, you can figure out if you're ready to give kickboxing a try.

It can be a very good way to lose the weight you need to lose. You can burn up to 450 calories in 30 minutes, making it a really great workout. It targets your upper body, lower body, and the core. This definitely is great on your cardiovascular system and will improve your lung capacity as time goes on. If you have a well-rounded set of workouts within kickboxing, your body will round itself out pretty easily. Kickboxing is a wonderful idea to help you lose weight and tone your body.

Rowing

Rowing is another intense workout, burning up to 660 calories per hour, but it is also easy to learn and is usually accessible through your local gym's rowing machines. You may want to ask a staff member before you try out the rowing machine to make sure that you use it properly. Also, keep in mind that this exercise is deceptively intense: it starts out feeling pretty low-key, but the muscle burn will set in pretty quickly. It is best to start out doing the exercise for only 10 to 15 minutes, and you can work your way up from there.

This machine targets your legs and butt, specifically the quads and upper thighs, along with the calves and glutes. This is what makes the workout so intense. Your shoulders, triceps, biceps, back, and core also get a workout. It's a low-impact workout, but that doesn't mean it's easy. With all of the muscle groups that are getting worked, it's not hard to see how it can be incredibly difficult to do.

This is a workout that anyone can do. It was actually originally made for anyone, including people aged 10 to 94 and people who were overweight and unable to do other workouts. It's not hard to learn how to properly do this, and it is something you can do for a long time. It slowly gets easier as long as you push through it to the very end.

Rowing, as a sport, is very collaborative. Therefore, it makes sense that you might work with other people and all row together, even on an indoor machine. You can get into a team mentality and be more collaborative with others. This machine is completely about resistance. How much you put into the machine in terms of resistance will determine how hard it will be. The harder you push and pull the machine, the harder it will be to do, and the more resistance you will have.

Rowing is a wonderful muscle building and weight loss workout. You'll feel the burn quickly and continue to feel like you are really working to do exactly what you want to do. The fat and calories will burn right off the more often you do it, making this a great exercise for anyone.

Elliptical Trainers

Elliptical trainers are a great way to start out your fitness journey because they are easy to use properly, and you can start out slowly and work your way up while using the same machine throughout. Ellipticals, as with treadmills, will also let you monitor your speed, heart rate, and certain other data to make sure that you are getting an efficient and effective workout. They are a great alternative to treadmills and to running outside because they provide a very low-impact workout while still allowing for a good deal of intensity.

Your local gym will almost certainly provide elliptical trainers because they are one of the most popular exercise machines out there. If you discover that you really like the elliptical and it is in your budget, you could also purchase your own for those days when you might not have the time or inclination to go out to the gym. You do not need a commercial-level elliptical to get a great workout.

Ellipticals are universal. People can use them in all stages of life, as long as they aren't injured. Some people feel a sense of security from the easy gliding motion that an elliptical provides. It's also incredibly easy to use.

All these activities have several things in common. One of these things is that they help burn calories and reduce weight through unconventional workout methods. Another important thing in common for all these activities would be the benefits to the cardiovascular system. Aside from working your abs or biceps and triceps, an important aspect of healthy living is a healthy heart and lungs. Fresh air and spending time with your friends contribute to healthy living as well, because a healthy body is useless without a healthy mind. Not all exercises need to be expensive because nature provides you with the opportunity for a cheap yet very beneficial workout – sometimes even more beneficial than a gym workout.

Whether or not you decide to take on some of these activities, you need to know that you don't have to spend a lot of money for gym membership or equipment in order to have a healthy lifestyle. The possibilities are endless because nature provides you with the best possible gym you would ever want or need. Health should not be a serious money-making business. You are able to figure out on your own what exercises will work best for you and will allow you to achieve your fitness and weight loss goals.

Nicholas Bjorn

Chapter 17: Exercise Your Body And Your Mind – The Benefits Of Yoga

In recent years, alternative ways of exercising are gaining more and more popularity. This movement includes some types of exercise that were introduced to the widespread audience through cultures that have survived for thousands of years. One of the most popular alternative ways of training that became popular is yoga.

Yoga can be described as a combination of spiritual and mental exercises, as well as physical exercise. With yoga, the benefits that your body reap are not only limited to your body. Your mind and your soul are able to find much-needed peace and serenity. Yoga's origins go back to ancient India, where it was practiced by monks who saw it as more than just an exercise for the body.

Recently, western cultures have put yoga through the eyes of science, trying to figure out how exactly yoga affects the body. What scientists found was that yoga helps the human body become healthy or recover from some injuries by alleviating the pain, aside from many other benefits.

If we are to look at the benefits of practicing yoga, we will end up with a long list that has to do with both the body and mind. Some of these benefits include: increased flexibility, stronger muscles, improved posture, boosting immunity, losing weight, increased blood flow, elevated heart beat rate, protection of the spine and other bones in the body, and many others.

Increased Flexibility

When talking about the benefits of yoga, among the first benefits that come to mind is increased flexibility. After the first training session, you probably would not be able to touch your toes or perform some other little more physically demanding activity, but after some time, you will be amazed at the effect of yoga on your flexibility. Activities that were a problem for you in the past will become as easy as waving a hand after a certain number of yoga sessions. Moreover, you will be very surprised with what your body can do. You will also be amazed at the disappearance of back pain and soreness of your muscles as you continue with the yoga sessions. One of the good consequences of the increased flexibility of your body is improved posture. The longer you keep up performing yoga, the more flexible you'll find your body to be. There will likely be a day when you can do a yoga pose you never thought you'd be able to do. This is all because you stuck with it, and your body listened to everything yoga was helping it do.

Improved Posture

Given that one of the crucial notions in yoga is balance, the improved posture of your body is no surprise. When you start with a yoga workout, which forces you to keep your head balanced directly over the spine and a way that takes the pressure from your neck and your shoulder. Thus, keeping your head straight becomes easier because the weight is now distributed through the spine and not on your neck and shoulders only. In case the weight of the head is not distributed through the entire spine, your neck and shoulders are under constant pressure, which may result in neck and shoulder pain, as well as back problems. One of the consequences of bad posture is chronic fatigue. Improving your posture through yoga will make your body feel less tired and ready for new tasks.

Back Pain Treatment

Related to its effect on posture, yoga can also be an effective treatment for chronic back pain. In fact, studies have shown that for many people, yoga can be more effective in treating chronic back pain than standard treatment options.

Yoga helps with back pain in several ways. The stretching and relaxation that occurs as a natural side effect of yoga help the back muscles and the spine to relax, thus decreasing stress to the area. Yoga also enhances blood flow, which lets essential nutrients into the back and allows toxins to flow out. Finally, yoga allows for the strengthening of muscles, which provides more support to the back when spinal issues are involved.

Stronger Muscles

Although there is no heavy weight lifting or amazingly hard chin-ups, pull-ups, or other muscle-building exercises, yoga provides you with the opportunity to do exactly that – make your muscles stronger. Surprisingly, yoga is also one of the best ways to make your muscles leaner and stronger. If we disregard the visual effects of lean and strong muscles, the medical reasons for those types of muscle will make you want to go and work on your muscles. With the benefits of stronger muscles, such as protection against certain diseases like back pain or arthritis, it is no wonder that many world-famous athletes incorporate yoga into their workout regimes.

Losing Weight

Just like any other physical activity out there, yoga helps reduce your body weight. A lot of people wonder how yoga can help in that aspect, as it is surprising how much it affects body weight. Although it may seem that there is not a lot of physical activity for losing weight, the number of calories burned during a yoga session can be comparable to that burned during physically active workouts. Of course, having only a yoga workout is not enough to lose weight. However, the combination of healthy diet, controlled caloric intake, and yoga workouts can do wonders for your body. Yoga may not be as effective as cross-country skiing, swimming, or running, but with it, you get something that you cannot get from any other activity from this list. What is unique for yoga is the fact that it provides you with spiritual satisfaction as well.

Increased Blood Flow AND Elevated Heart Beat Rate

One of the great benefits of a yoga workout can be seen in the blood flow and heartbeat rate. Some of the relaxing exercises included in a yoga workout improve blood circulation in your body. After a yoga workout, you will feel much better because yoga enables the cells of your body to intake more oxygen, which results in improved health. Certain exercises, such as a headstand or handstand, enable the blood from the lower parts of your body to go through the heart and lungs, where it will get fresh oxygen and thus provide you with more energy. On the other hand, some yoga exercises that can be described as aerobic increase your heart rate in such a way that it can reduce the risk of heart attack, as well as help fight against depression.

Boosting Immunity

One of the main conditions for your body to stay healthy is for its immune system to be properly working. Yoga does exactly that – it boosts your immune system to a level that the body is able to fight all kinds of viruses and bacteria that are potentially dangerous. Given that a yoga workout includes muscle stretching and even moving your organs around, your lymph system becomes more active, and as it becomes more active, the number of immune cells in your body increases, which results in stronger immunity to certain diseases, viruses, or bacteria. From the medical point of view, this lymph system is in charge of fighting against all kinds of infection, as well as against certain types of cancerous cells, so why wouldn't you want to boost the system that keeps your healthy and safe your entire life?

Improved Mental Health

It is well-established that exercise can help with depression and anxiety, among other mental health concerns, and yoga is no exception to that rule. In fact, yoga has been shown to be of benefit to individuals living with schizophrenia, depression, sleep problems, and other psychiatric conditions. In addition to the usual benefits of exercise, the focus on community and cooperation that takes place in yoga classes stimulates your body's production of oxytocin and serotonin, both of which help to combat the negative symptoms of depression and other mental health issues.

Increasing Fertility And The Likelihood Of Pregnancy

While the practice of yoga does not directly impact one's fertility, the relaxing and de-stressing effect of yoga can increase the chances of conceiving by improving blood flow to the body, including the reproductive organs. In addition, it is well-known that stress can be an impediment to conceiving, so stress reduction alone could improve the situation.

Hangover Cure

While we have already talked earlier in this book about the fact that it is best to avoid alcohol if you really want to improve your fitness levels, there may be the occasion where you decide to indulge. If you do, yoga can help you the next day, when you wake up and are not feeling particularly well. Certain poses, such as the plow, shoulder stand, and fish, work to boost the thyroid gland's function and improve metabolism, which will work the toxins out of your system more quickly.

Easing Asthma Symptoms

Studies have shown that the regular practice of yoga can drastically reduce asthma symptoms. This is partly because of the overall physical benefits of yoga, in that a healthier and fitter body will naturally have better lung function, but also because yoga focuses so much on breathing practice, which in itself helps to combat asthma symptoms.

Fighting Arthritis

Iyengar yoga in particular – a type of yoga that incorporates props, such as blocks, belts, and other positioning aids – has been shown to be helpful to people who are living with rheumatoid arthritis. Other types of yoga, such as Bikram, can help because the heat involved makes it easier for the body to go through the movements. If practiced properly, most forms of yoga will provide some benefit to individuals experiencing arthritis, because the gentle movements can allow for individuals to practice yoga when other types of exercise may be too hard on their bodies.

Better Sleep

In addition to the general stress-reducing aspects of yoga, which can help improve your sleep patterns, there are specific yoga movements that, if done before bed, can help you fall asleep more easily. The forward fold, or forward bend, is one such pose: sit on the floor with your legs straight out in front of you. Inhale and lift your arms up over your head, lengthening through your torso up through the crown of your head and your fingers. While exhaling, hinge at the hips, and slowly lower your torso toward your legs. Reach toward your ankles, feet, or toes as you are able. If you want to deepen the stretch, you can use your arms to gently pull your torso closer to your legs. Once you are in position, breathe and hold the position for 3 to 8 breaths, then slowly roll your spine back up until you are in the seated position.

Another very simple exercise is to lie on your back with your legs and feet against the wall. This basic position helps with circulation and relaxing your body.

Combating Multiple Sclerosis Symptoms

Some of the frustrating symptoms of multiple sclerosis include loss of coordination and muscle function. While yoga can by no means cure or prevent multiple sclerosis, it can help reduce the worsening of symptoms by improving the body's overall function.

Dealing With PTSD

Perhaps not too surprisingly, given the other benefits discussed above, recent studies have shown that yoga may assist individuals who are living with PTSD. The improved physical and mental functions offered by yoga could provide assistance to these individuals and may be especially helpful to people who have not found success with more traditional treatments, such as psychotherapy.

As we have seen in this part about yoga, it is evident that the benefits of yoga workout remain desirable for almost all humans. Given that yoga was used in ancient times by Buddhist monks, it is evident that the benefits of yoga overcome the body and move into the sphere of the spiritual, and we all know how important peace of mind is. Unlike many other activities mentioned here, yoga is far from being fast-moving, and that is exactly the point of yoga exercises. Yoga strips you of everyday worries and responsibilities and provides you with the opportunity to meditate, relax, and exercise in peace and silence and to fully devote your attention to your body and the needs of your body.

Given that there are many types of yoga, be sure to find the one type that suits you and your needs the most. Sometimes, the wrong type of exercise can do much more damage than good. Many physical activities are not recommended for people who have some heart problems, diabetes, high blood pressure, or arthritis. However, people with these kinds of problems are encouraged to take on yoga because it can help them with those problems. Even if you are pregnant, yoga is probably the best choice for you because it will help you become more relaxed and strong during the pregnancy period.

Chapter 18: Make Your Own Gym At Home

If you don't want to constantly spend money on a gym membership or to exercise in crowded gyms, but you still would want to exercise, this section will provide you with some ideas for doing exactly that. For those who can afford the items, the following list will definitely prove to be useful in daily exercising and keeping your body healthy. If your income allows you to spend a certain amount of money on home gym equipment, you will be able to have a daily exercising regimen right in your home.

With these ideas on how to make your own gym at your own home, you can have exactly what your body wants and needs. Whether you want to exercise your muscles, increase your muscle strength, or do some cardio exercises, the list below provides you with the best equipment to do just that. The following equipment will provide you with the opportunity to work on your muscles, flexibility, cardio, and strength.

A Punching Bag

When you come home after the hard day at work, you might sometimes just want to hit somebody. Well, a punching bag provides you with the opportunity to do that. A workout session on the punching bag is one of the best cardio workouts that can be done with the equipment mentioned in this part. The workout that you will be doing with a punching bag will help you be in shape, increase the strength of your body, make your muscles leaner, as well as burn a good amount of calories while relieving all of your stress. Another benefit of a punching bag that must be mentioned is the opportunity for you to develop your self-defense abilities, which can be crucial at some point in your life. A workout on a punching bag will also help be more balanced and coordinated. What must be noted here are, once again, the notion of the proper use of the equipment and the notion of pre-warm up. One of the greatest benefits of a punching bag is the amount of money you need to spend to set up such equipment in comparison to similar workout sessions in the gym. On that note, a solid-quality punching bag can be obtained at Amazon for $89.99.

Punching bags can help you work out your entire body. If you want a specific workout to follow, kickboxing and regular boxing are great ones to look at. However, if you just want to have something to punch, owning a punching bag will be extremely beneficial. So many things will be improved, including your power, aerobic fitness, coordination, core strength, and even your boxing technique. When using a punching bag, the main muscles you use are going to be in the upper body. The shoulders, arms, back, chest, and waist will constantly be used, which will help you stay in shape and shed off the pounds. Depending on what kinds of jabs you do, you will work those muscles in different ways. Investing in a punching bag means you'll be able to see your body transform in front of you. You can always destress after a particularly long day of work, which is something everyone wants to do at one point or another. As long as you stick to the proper techniques and always prepare properly, you'll have great progress with a punching bag.

An Elliptical Machine

One of the best benefits of an elliptical machine is the fact that it enables you to have low-impact workout sessions. These kinds of sessions are very important for people who have certain health issues, such as heart conditions or back pain. For those people, equipment like this provides them with the opportunity to work out, repair their injuries, and burn calories in a way that is adjusted to their body limitations. An elliptical machine is a great opportunity to work your arm and leg muscles, as well as to increase the strength of your body in general. Moreover, a workout on an elliptical machine will improve coordination between your hands and legs, as well as the throughout your body. Elliptical machines are also very effective in helping you recover from injuries and boosting your immune system because the effort put in the exercise on this equipment is not too hard for an injured body to handle but still intense enough to boost your heart beat rate. Furthermore, this type of machine will enable you to multitask because it will allow you to watch a movie or your favorite cooking show while still exercising. As regards the cost, it must be noted that the price is not one of the advantages as it is one of the costliest among the equipment in this section. That being said, an elliptical machine can be bought at Amazon for $1,169.97.

The elliptical is a great machine for people with many different body types, young or old. It provides a low-impact workout, making it easy on the joints and on your body in general while still being a huge calorie burner. At the same time, there isn't any weight bearing element to it like there is on a treadmill, so you won't get the same bone and muscle strengthening as you would with a treadmill. If you have bad joints, then an elliptical is definitely the first choice you should consider. Some people have found the elliptical boring or not challenging enough, but it can do so much more than people seem to give it credit for. This piece of equipment is great because it doesn't just provide a leg workout: it provides an arm workout, too. Of course, you need to use the bars if you want it to definitely work your upper body. Another phenomenal thing about the elliptical is that you don't always have to go forward. You can actually reverse your movements and go backwards, which gives your quads a much bigger workout.

Another great benefit is that an elliptical is highly sought after as a way to bounce back from injuries. After you get doctor's approval, an elliptical might be a great way to get full motion back in your knee, ankle, or hips. It works all of these areas to some extent, strengthening them and making them better than they were before the injury. On top of that, there's also the fun part where it's easy to multitask on an elliptical. Maybe there's a TV show or a movie you really want to watch. Maybe you have a book that you're close to finishing. The elliptical is a great way to be able to do just that. Overall, an elliptical is a great choice for so many different reasons, but it's up to you if it's right for your needs.

A Treadmill

One of the most typical equipment for exercising is the treadmill. Being one of the main elements of every gym, a treadmill is also one of the most popular exercise equipment. Running is healthy. Running in nature is healthier. However, if you don't have the opportunity to run in nature, or weather conditions are not allowing such an activity, a treadmill will be a great choice if you need to stay indoors and still do some exercise. One of the advantages of using a treadmill in your exercise regimen is the fact that you, as a user, can control the way in which you run. What this means is that you are able to control the speed of the run, how much resistance you want, and other elements. Additionally, some treadmills have step counters, which provide you with the opportunity to monitor what distance you have run. There are also counters for burned calories with the same purpose. Just like ordinary running, a treadmill enables you to burn calories, as well as increase your heart rate or blood flow and the level of oxygen in the cardiovascular system. Running on a treadmill has another advantage, and that is multitasking. While running on a treadmill, you are still able to watch your favorite TV show while exercising.

However, treadmills also have certain disadvantages. One of these is the fact that the maintenance of the device is too complicated for the common user, so a professional has to do the maintaining, and that can sometimes cause certain problems. Another problem related to treadmills is their size. In the majority of cases, they occupy a lot of space, so a pre-condition of buying a treadmill is securing enough space. One of the most crucial disadvantages of treadmills is their price. You can purchase a treadmill at Amazon within the price range of $999 to $2,000.

The treadmill is a great choice for those who want a lot of versatility in the way they run. Maybe it's your first time running. You'll be able to set your treadmill at lower settings. Maybe you want it to be very challenging. You can set it on a hill or at a faster rate, making it much harder on the body. You can definitely lose some weight on a treadmill. While it's always a good idea to vary your workouts, if you spend 40 minutes on a treadmill everyday amidst your other workouts, then you'll easily notice a change in your body. Given that a treadmill is more demanding on your body, you'll actually burn a lot more calories than you might burn otherwise.

Treadmills are also one of the most researched workout equipment out there, so they have been modified and improved in many different ways. These are especially good for those who enjoy walking and running compared to other workouts. While you'll still need to complete other workouts in order to get your body in the shape you want, you can definitely have the treadmill as your main cardio source.

Medicine Balls

All the equipment mentioned so far comprised machine equipment. However, all exercise equipment does not need to be mechanical in order to be functional and beneficial for your health and body. One piece of such equipment is a medicine ball. Medicine balls are often used by professional athletes because they improve endurance, strength, coordination, and flexibility, along with many other benefits. The history of the medicine balls goes back to ancient times. In ancient Greece, medicine balls were used by healers in order to improve the recovery of patients who sustained certain types of injuries. Unlike many other types of equipment, medicine balls are suitable for everyone. People of all ages are able to use them in their workout. There are several sizes of medicine balls, starting from 2 pounds to 12 pounds, so they are suitable even for children. One of the most important advantages of medicine balls is the fact that they help improve the strength of abdominal region, as well as the spine and the lower and upper back.

The most important concept related to medicine balls is motion. In order to enjoy the benefits of medicine balls, your body must be in motion while using them. Whether it be by moving your torso from side to side while holding medicine balls in your hands, throwing medicine balls up against the wall and catching them, or having someone throw you a medicine ball while you try to catch it, medicine balls seem to be one of the best non-mechanical piece of equipment used for exercise. Moreover, medicine balls are often used in the rehabilitation process. If you, by any chance, have injured a shoulder, medicine balls would be a great choice for recovery. One way in which you could use medicine balls in this case is to take a 2-pound medicine ball, stand next to the wall, throw the medicine ball against the wall using the hand on the side of your injured shoulder, raise your arm above your head, and try to catch the ball as it comes back. The injured shoulder is used to throw the medicine ball against the wall. It is also important to emphasize that before taking up medicine balls for exercise, pre-warm up is crucial. Otherwise, you risk getting injuries or making an already existing injury worse. It is important also to mention that the price of this equipment is not that high, as it can be purchased at Amazon for $59.11.

Using a medicine ball is also a great thing to do with a friend, which will make it a great workout. There are so many different workouts you can do with a partner, but one of them is the sit-up pass. With this, each person lays with ankles in line with each other. One has the medicine ball, and you both sit up. The one with the medicine ball passes it to the other person, and then you both lay back down. The faster you can do this exercise without going too fast that you lose control, the more of a workout you'll be able to get. Working with a partner is always a great idea with something like this, since you'll both be in motion, even when you don't have the medicine ball in your hands.

Medicine balls are great because of the different weights you can choose from. You can start out with a lower weight, and as you progress, you can increase the weights. Many gyms will have medicine balls up to twenty or thirty pounds. If you would like to get higher weighted medicine balls, then look for them online. Medicine balls can add a lot to your daily workout. If you do many reps with a lower weight, just like with any weightlifting regimen, you'll be able to slowly build the muscle you want without needing a machine to help you.

A Jump Rope

Not all pieces of equipment for exercise need to be expensive or technically sophisticated. Some of them can be as simple as a rope. This is exactly the case with a jump role – no sophisticated programs, no hardware, no software, and no cables – just plain and simple rope. Although it may seem like a child's game, a jump role is actually pretty effective in burning calories and losing weight. A jump rope exercise will burn 480 calories in half an hour of training. Ten minutes spent exercising with a jump rope has the same effect as a 30-minute running session. Jumping rope in several sets will improve your body coordination like few other pieces of exercise equipment. Jumping rope is often performed by professional athletes, such as footballers, boxers, tennis players, basketball players, and many others for a quick cardio exercise that boosts their blood flow and increases their heart beat rate. One of the reasons why professional athletes use jump rope is the fact that such exercise helps with the recovery of a previously sustained foot or ankle injury. One of the best advantages of a jump rope is its size. Being small in size, it is possible to bring it with your wherever you go. Consequently, this means that you don't have to miss a workout even if you are traveling because you can bring your jump rope with you in your bag. Surprisingly, jump rope exercises also affect the brain's cognitive functions because they incorporate three elements (coordination, rhythm, and strategic organization) into an exercise plan. One of the best advantages of a jump rope is its price. It is one of the most affordable pieces of equipment for exercise that you can find on the market. It can be purchased at Amazon for only $14.97.

Another great thing about a jump rope is that it can really power up your speed levels. If you get a regular jump rope, there's a great possibility that you'll be able to go faster than you ever thought you could. If you want a little more of a challenge, though, you can buy a weighted jump rope. This will allow you to gain some muscle through this simple exercise. Moreover, your endurance levels will go way up. Having a weight on something that is meant to be moved quickly helps your body be ready for unexpected things. Weighted jump ropes are also good for losing weight. They are specifically made with the idea of burning calories in mind. This means that if you are really into losing some weight, a weighted jump rope might just be what's right for you. This will allow you to shed off the pounds by mixing a jump rope with your usual workout routine. In no time, you'll be marveling at how you managed to become the person you wanted to be.

Ab Wheel

Another pretty affordable piece of exercise equipment is the ab wheel. An ab wheel is a small wheel that has two handles on either side. This piece of equipment can be purchased at Amazon for $28. Although exercises performed with the ab wheel may seem to require little effort from the user, the reality is totally different. You might have a problem in the beginning when you start to use the ab wheel, unless you already possess a powerful core and well-balanced body. One of the best advantages of this piece of equipment is that when you use it, your spine returns to a natural position, and your muscles get well-balanced. A natural position of your spine means good posture for your body and, consequently, a healthier spine and bones. When you use the ab wheel correctly, your body uses several muscles in order to push the wheel away and bring it closer. Exercising with an ab wheel involves more than 20 muscles. If you want eye-turning abs and, more importantly, a healthy body, you might use the ab wheel because the parts of your body that exert the most effort are the abdominal muscles. The ab wheel is also a very good piece of equipment for burning calories and losing weight. It is small in size, so you can bring it with you on your travels, which makes it one of only a few pieces of equipment that are portable. You should be very careful when using this equipment because if it is used in the wrong way, it may result in certain injuries.

Although there are many advantages of an ab wheel, it also has several disadvantages. The most important disadvantage is the amount of pressure that this kind of exercise places on your lower back. If the muscles of your lower back and hips are not strong enough, it is possible that this exercise may result in pain or even injury.

It's very important to know how to use an ab wheel properly. Again, improper use can lead to injury, which is the last thing you want when trying to be in shape or to lose weight. In order to use this device properly, you need to follow these steps: Place the ab wheel below your shoulders, latching onto the handles, and having your arms and back straight. From there, roll the wheel forward slowly. Make sure to keep your core tightened and your back straight, as these will reduce the chances of any injury. Once you get to the furthest point you can while still keeping your body straight, move back using your core. Be sure not to use your hips to move back, as this will completely negate all of the work you've tried to do. This is the basic ab wheel exercise that will get your abs working. If your abs are not very strong, this will likely be a difficult thing to start doing. Patience is needed here. Eventually, you will be able to do the things you've always wanted to do. If you become too impatient and try to do things before you should, this will end in disaster. However, if you stick with the plan, then things can work out in your favor.

Kettlebell

The kettlebell is a piece of exercise equipment that looks similar to a cannonball but with a handle on it. Kettlebells come in a variety of weights and are quite inexpensive. Exercises performed with kettlebells combine cardiovascular, flexibility, and strength training, and they are easy to learn and to perform properly.

The benefit of kettlebell exercises is that they tend to work several key muscle groups at a time, which means that these exercises fall more under interval training than traditional weightlifting despite the fact that it may look like lifting weights. Kettlebell exercises tend to involve multiple repetitions, but beginners should start out slowly and focus on doing the exercises properly rather than achieving high numbers of repetitions.

Kettlebell exercises offer improved range of motion, mobility, and strength, but should be avoided by people who have shoulder or back problems. They can be as cheap as $8 on Amazon, making them a great thing to add to your equipment. Given that they are such an inexpensive device to add to your equipment, you can buy them in many different weights and add them to your medicine ball collection. You can also opt to go with kettlebells instead of medicine balls.

Kettlebells are very interesting, and they really keep you in good health. They can strengthen your tendons and ligaments, which in turn makes your joints stronger. They are used in a different ways than medicine balls, which is something some people aren't aware of. Obviously, this means that anyone can use kettlebells. They may look intimidating, but they are much more helpful than you may think they would be. Given that they come in many sizes, someone who is a little older and who might have some joint pain can grab a lighter kettlebell and slowly work his or her way up to a heavier one. This way, this person will be able to slowly add onto the weight he or she has been carrying.

Overall, kettlebells are a great investment to your home gym. Given that they work different muscles than the medicine ball, you can have a few of each and use them interchangeably. Adding some kettlebells can make your workout a more comprehensive one than it might normally be. Of course, this means you have to keep up with the workout. Doing it for a few days and then stopping won't change anything, but if you keep at it, you'll likely change your body significantly.

Free Weights

If you have kettlebells and medicine balls, why do you still need free weights? Well, these weights work different muscles in your arms than the others do. Free weights come in as light as 2 pounds and as heavy as 80 pounds at a gym, though they do go higher if you want to purchase them. You can also buy adjustable free weights, where you can add weight onto the ends, making them even heavier. Those can go up to 200 pounds.

For those who might not know, a free weight refers to the stereotypical weights you usually see people using. They come in a set, each weighing, say, five pounds. They are basically like a bar with a weight on either end, but miniaturized to fit in your hands. These are incredibly useful when you're trying to build up lean muscles. Moreover, you don't need to have a spotter if you use these. That being said, you need to be careful when using them, especially as the weight goes up. Using them improperly can lead to an injury that might be hard to recover from.

Using free weights forces your muscles to work together, eventually creating balance. There are some exercises you could do to focus on one or maybe two muscles and nothing else. This can be very counterproductive if you are trying to balance your body out. As free weights are, well, free, you can not only so many different things with them, but it's also what helps you build lean muscle and give your body a more balanced look. There are tons of free weights available to buy at local stores and online. On Amazon in particular, you can start with a set of 3, 5, or 8 free weights for only $45. While it is a bit of an investment, it will pay off in the future.

These weights are great for burning calories. They really target muscles in order to strengthen them. You could do a full body workout and burn even more calories, all while strengthening your muscles. Of course, one of the best things about free weights, especially if you buy them for your home gym, is that they can be put away very easily. They are very easy to move and put into a closet or on a rack, which is something that will come in handy as you get more weights. Free weights are incredibly versatile, which means that there are tons of ways to use them. The sheer magnitude of exercises for people using free weights is astounding. They range from simple bicep curls to something that will make you use muscles throughout your entire body. There are endless possibilities, which is why free weights would make a great addition to your home gym.

Exercise (Yoga) Mat

While yoga and other floor exercises do not require an exercise mat, these mats can be very helpful if you are doing this kind of activity. The mats are designed to provide enough cushion to safeguard you from the soreness that comes from working out on a hardwood or tile floor or other hard surfaces, but not so much cushioning that it reduces the effect of the exercises that you are doing.

Along with the cushioning, it can give you a solid, comfortable surface to do your exercises on. Without a yoga mat, you could slip and fall or just feel completely uncomfortable with all of your exercises. The great thing about an exercise mat is that it isn't only for doing yoga. It's also for doing other exercises that require you to stand for long periods of time or those that need a good, solid surface to stand or move on. A yoga mat is just a great accessory to have, especially in a home gym.

Foam Roller

The foam roller is not a piece of exercise equipment, but it does come in very handy after working out because it is a fantastic way to roll out tight and sore muscles. It is basically a way of giving yourself a massage, but the benefit of the foam roller is that it makes it very easy to do the process properly and avoid causing an injury. By applying pressure to certain points on your body, particularly the areas that you just targeted in your workout, you can improve muscle recovery.

The foam roller works best when used on trigger points, which are knots that form in your muscles. These areas are easily identified because they will feel painful when you put pressure on them. If you roll a trigger point (such as in your calf) over the foam roller, it will gradually break up the muscle knots and allow normal blood flow to return to the area. Keep in mind that this will hurt at first because you are applying pressure to those knots. As you continue to use the foam roller, you will note that the pain gradually decreases as the knot is worked out, and blood flow returns.

Foam rollers may seem silly, but they can be so beneficial. Everyone who's had a sore back in their life know that the pain can make it nearly impossible to concentrate on the things they need to, especially if you go to the gym semi-regularly. There are, of course, days that you should simply take off and res. These days might make you realize just how sore your back is because it hasn't been worked in a few days or because it was worked in ways it hasn't been worked before. These muscles need some sort of release from the agony they are in, and a foam roller can give the release you desire. A foam roller will be a great investment that can give you everything you need after a hard day at the gym.

Resistance Bands

Resistance bands, also known as exercise bands, are a very useful tool for strength training and general fitness exercises. Some of the exercises included in the earlier chapters this book involve the use of resistance bands. Resistance bands are usually purchased in sets, with different colors used to indicate increasing levels of resistance. Beginners should start with the lowest resistance and work their way up as their fitness improves.

An advantage of resistance bands is that they are very lightweight, and they fold up into a very small package, making them a great option to bring with you when you are traveling and want to make sure that you can still get a workout in.

Resistance bands can be combined with other exercises to increase difficulty, and there are exercises that can be done specifically with the resistance bands. Most resistance band kits will even come with a few suggested exercises that you can use to start out with. You can get a starter kit on Amazon for $20, which will give you a few different bands, a door anchor, an ankle strap, an exercise chart, and a carrying case for your resistance bands.

Resistance bands have tons of benefits. They not only make your muscles and bones stronger but also work parts of your body that are harder to target. They can also help improve your balance, reduce joint pain, improve your speed of movement, and make your body more elastic. No, that doesn't mean that your body will suddenly move in weird ways that you didn't think were possible, but it will mean that your movements will be more fluid. You'll have the strength to help your body do the things it needs to do.

You don't need to have a partner to use a resistance band. If you want to work your legs, if you have a door anchor and an ankle strap, you'll be golden. Moreover, these definitely are a great thing to add in after you've already been working out. It will add a variety to your workout, catching your body off guard. It will increase your stamina and add to your range of motion.

Exercise Videos

Buying exercise videos to work out with at home is a great way to add variety to your daily workout. For some people, having a pre-made routine to follow improves the likelihood that they will work out; for others, it is nice to have a cardio option available when the weather outside is not great. The benefit of videos is that they do not usually require specialized equipment, or if they do, it is usually equipment that is easy to get and fairly inexpensive, such as resistance bands or free weights.

There are so many different types of workouts available on video that there is something for virtually everyone: Zumba, kickboxing, step aerobics – you name it, there is a video for it. If you are not sure what kind of exercise will work best for you, you can try and see if there are videos online of the different exercises so that you can try them out first before purchasing your own, or your local gym might have some available to borrow.

Exercise videos are especially helpful when you are just starting out. Maybe you don't feel comfortable going to the gym yet, and you'd rather start at home, doing something you think might be fun. You can start the road to getting the body you want and do it all in the comfort of your home. Going to the gym can be intimidating, especially at first, but it can be less intimidating if you start at home first. Of course, you could grow to love exercise videos and decide you'd rather workout to these at home. You'll need to make sure to have some other types of equipment around if you want to do that, as you need to have some variety to what you do. This will keep your body guessing at what you might do next and thus help it evolve. Maybe doing two days of a Zumba video and one day of weights would work. Anything you might think would work for what you want your body to be is what you should go with.

Just remember that, as with any exercise that you are doing, it is important to focus on doing the exercises properly rather than always keeping up with what is happening in the video. If you are starting out in more of a beginner position than the video provides for, just do what you can, and make sure that you do not push yourself too hard or you will risk injury.

As we have seen throughout this book, paying huge gym membership fees in order for you to remain in shape and to exercise your body and your mind is not the only solution. It is possible to have all the effects of gym sessions from the comfort of your own home. Making a gym at home by buying certain pieces of equipment should be done according to plan based on the needs and requirements of your body. Although some exercise equipment may be beyond the price range of common people, there are some that are cheap but with the same or even better effects than the more expensive ones. The risk of injury is present with every piece of exercise equipment, so you should be extra careful if you are using these elements for exercising, especially if you are working out alone.

Chapter 19: The Importance Of Water For The Human Body

Although water is a crucial element in sustaining life on Earth, many of us fail to recognize how important water is for the human body and what devastating effects the lack of water consumption can have on our health. Given that the human body is composed of more than 50% water, it is really unbelievable how some people just disregard this fact. Without water, there is no life, and without water in the human body, it is impossible for the body to perform its functions in a proper way. Humans are capable of surviving several days without any food, but when it comes to water, the human body is only capable of surviving a few days before shutting down permanently.

Every single cell of the human body uses water in order to regulate cell temperature. Although some experts claim that there is a certain amount of water that every person should drink every day, there are also those who claim that water intake depends on several factors. Some of these factors are the climate in your location, how much do you exercise, how much you weigh, you age, and several others. As regards the amount of water every person should drink on a daily basis, the number differs for every person, but many agree that it should be between 2 and 2.5 liters of water per day. However, both of these groups of experts agree on the following: Water is crucial in maintaining a healthy body. To preserve the health of our body, we have a duty to drink enough water. Our body uses water for the removal of dangerous elements from our organs through sweating, urination, and other body functions.

Every human organ demands a certain amount of water. However, three areas that are affected the most by the lack of water intake are the brain, blood, and muscles. Notably, 85% of the human brain is made up of the water, and the lack of water strongly influences our brain, which can result in terrible headaches or other more dangerous consequences. Headaches caused by the lack of water sometimes transform into a migraine, a terrible headache for which scientists have not yet found a cure. Given that a migraine results in terrible pain, the human body is forced to shut down certain functions, which is one of the reasons why people feel dehydrated, tired, and exhausted after the pain of a migraine has passed. Moreover, the lack of water in the human brain can result in such problems as short-term memory, inability to solve simple mathematical problems, as well as issues with concentration.

On the other hand, human blood is made up of 80% of water. Blood, being one of the crucial elements in the human body, is then strongly affected by the lack of water. Given that blood is responsible for maintaining the health of our brain, the lack of water poses a serious threat to our health. Blood that is affected by the lack of water is not able to protect our body, which consequently gets infected by many kinds of viruses or bacteria. Weak blood means a weak body. It has also been proven that the lack of water can lead to high blood pressure and all the problems that come with it.

The muscles of the human body are 70% water. In trying to build stronger and better looking muscles, we often forget to consume enough water. In order to maintain a certain level of muscle strength, it is necessary to consume water constantly. With the lack of water, muscles in the human body lose their strength, and consequently, the body becomes progressively weaker. As a consequence, the human body gets tired more quickly, it takes a longer time to fully relax, and coordination and balance become weaker.

Common Misconceptions

There are several misconceptions as regards water. One of the most prevalent is that certain types of drinks can replace water. Some people believe that such drinks as soft drinks, alcohol, tea, energy drinks, and coffee are an adequate replacement for water. However, no other drink has the same qualitative values as water. A bottle of soft drink cannot replace a bottle of water. Moreover, soft drinks are bad for your health because they contain sugar and other additives, which can have negative effects on your heart and blood pressure. Unlike water, soft drinks are unable to quench your thirst. What they actually do is they make you even thirstier than before, creating a cycle involving soft drinks, water, and thirst. Moreover, coffee and tea cannot be an adequate replacement for water, as they are actually diuretics. With the frequent intake of coffee or tea, your body loses the water that is required for its maintenance.

It is important to remember that sports drinks are also not a replacement for the water that your body needs. While sports drinks are useful in that they can replenish the electrolytes that your body may lose during high-intensity workouts during which you sweat a lot, they will not replenish your body's supply of water. Only drinking water will give your body the water that it needs to maintain its functions.

Energy drinks, unlike sports drinks, do not really provide any health benefit and are most definitely not a substitute for drinking water. Energy drinks tend to have very high levels of caffeine, which is why people drink them in the first place.

Some caffeine is beneficial, as it can boost your metabolism, but too much caffeine can cause an upset stomach, diarrhea, nervousness, and headaches. If you need some caffeine, try to stick with coffee, as its caffeine content is much lower than that of energy drinks.

Main Functions Of Water In The Human Body

If we were to write down all the functions of water in the human body, it would take a lot longer for this book to be published, and there would not be any foreseen deadline. Here, we will mention only a few of the most important functions of water in the human body. One of them is bringing oxygen and other nutrients to every possible cell. Without water, the cells in the human body would be rid of their food, and after some time, those cells would die out. Another important function of water is the regulation of temperature. Water in the human body maintains the optimum temperature, but if that system of protection is endangered by the lack of water, temperature can have devastating effects on the human body and your health. One of the crucial functions of water relative to the human body is related to the kidneys.

The function of the kidneys is to extract waste and other potentially dangerous elements from the human body through urination. In order for the kidneys to do their function, they require a sufficient amount of water. When water intake is insufficient, the kidneys will not be able to perform their function properly. In this case, waste and other potentially dangerous materials remain in the kidneys and other parts of the body. This can later cause serious health issues. Even the skin is affected by the lack of water. Water keeps human skin moist and healthy. The lack of water results in dry skin and other problems. There are many more functions of the water in the human body, but as previously mentioned, it will be almost impossible to list them all.

Water And Exercising

Drinking water is important, but drinking water before, while, or after a workout session at the gym, in nature, or at home is even more important. Exercising and other activities like watching TV or being at work are different in terms of how much effort it takes to perform them. Exercising is physically demanding activity, and as such, it results in much more sweat being lost. Consequently, exercising is an activity that demands a much bigger water intake. The problem with sweating as a result of exercise is the loss of not only water but also some other elements important to the proper functioning of the body. These elements need to be replaced, and the best way to do this is by drinking water. Water will replace lost elements in the majority of cases. However, in some cases, additional fluids will be necessary. Through sweating, we also lose electrolytes, which are important to replace, but water does not contain such elements. Some drinks, such as sports drinks and coconut water, contain these much-needed electrolytes and have been proven to be helpful in hydrating while working out. Another solution for the replacement of lost electrolytes is to eat fruits. However, not all fruits have the same amount of electrolytes. Bananas are an excellent choice as a source of electrolytes.

However, it is also important to drink some water even while eating fruits because, although fruits contain a certain amount of water, it is still not enough. One of the signs that your body is losing water and electrolytes and that it needs those elements to be replaced is when your muscles get easily tired. Even if you aren't exercising, you should definitely still be drinking plenty of water. Without water, you can easily become dehydrated, especially if you work out. Drinking water while working out is important, but it doesn't diminish the significance of drinking water when you're lounging at home and relaxing. This doesn't mean you shouldn't ever drink any other drink other than water; it just means that you need to be conscious of how much water you are consuming outside of your typical workouts.

Dehydration

Dehydration can be characterized as the lack of an adequate amount of fluid, mainly water, in the human body. There can be many reasons why dehydration occurs, that is, there are several ways in which body can lose such a large amount of fluid that it would lead to dehydration. Some of these reasons are frequent urination, diarrhea, or diabetes. Aside from these reasons, sweating and vomiting can lead to dehydration.

In professional sports, dehydration is a common thing because professional athletes exert so much effort that their bodies quickly lose fluids. However, when they are constantly consuming fluids, the balance in their bodies is maintained.

Dehydration is also a common state that occurs in intense workout sessions not only among the professional athletes but among common people as well. One difference between professional athletes and common people getting dehydrated through a workout is that professional athletes know the dangers of dehydration, and they have a team of people who look after them, so dehydration for them does not represent a real danger. On the other hand, common people do not really pay much attention to the amount of fluids consumed during a workout session, and because of that, they are in real danger of dehydration.

Dehydration occurs when the body has lost 2% of its total weight while doing exercise or some other related activity. When dehydration occurs, indicators of physical performance are reduced, heart beat rate often goes up, and a person loses the focus and coordination. Basically, dehydration occurs when the intake of water or other electrolyte-rich fluids is less than the amount of fluid lost through sweat during the workout session.

According to medical professionals, there are several signs that indicate that the body has come to a critical moment relative to the presence of fluids in the body. Some of those signs include a lack of sweat, small or negligible amount of urine, dark-colored urine, general weakness, dizziness, fatigue, dry mouth, dry skin, increased body temperature, elevated heart rate, constipation, headache, muscle cramps, and many others. Dehydration occurs more with such activities as running, swimming, and cycling than with such activities as lifting weights, chin-ups, or pull-ups because the former are much more demanding activities that causes the body to lose more fluids.

One of the consequences of dehydration is related to the kidneys and their function. With the lack of fluids in the body, it is possible for kidney stones to appear. This comes along with certain problems with the liver, muscles, and others. Dehydration does not only occur as a consequence of hard training or by being a professional athlete. Dehydration can also be symptom or consequence of some medical conditions, such as diarrhea or fever. People with these types of symptoms are much more prone to dehydration. One of the ways in which dehydration and all its effects can be avoided is to carry a bottle of water with you wherever you go. Regular intake of fluids, especially water, will replace the fluids lost through sweating, such that your body will not feel any consequence of the lack of water.

Some people believe that soft drinks are a good and adequate choice when faced with the challenge of choosing a replacement for the lost fluids during workout sessions. Soft drinks cannot replace water relative to dehydration. In order to overcome the effects of dehydration, a person must drink fluids that are rich in electrolytes. However, a large majority of soft drinks do not contain any electrolytes. Those that contain a certain amount of electrolytes often have added sugar as an ingredient, such that the effects of electrolytes are nullified. Often, after drinking soft drinks, your body feels even thirstier than it previously was. Thus, soft drinks must be avoided at any cost. If you are among those people who cannot stand the plain taste of water, there are several solutions for you. In this case, the best choice to replace the fluids in the body is by consuming juice made from freshly grown vegetables and fruits. However, you must be careful not to use too many fruits and vegetables because the juice might contain a lot of sugar and calories, which no longer make it healthy for your body.

Medical professionals keep reminding us that in order to stay healthy, we must drink enough water, and this is not only when we feel thirsty. Small sips of water should be taken during the entire day. A bottle of water must become first thing we grab when we go outside. In this way, we will prevent our body from becoming dehydrated so that we avoid all the dangerous effects that come with dehydration that can sometimes even be life-threatening.

Sufficient intake of fluids is crucial in keeping our body healthy and in shape. The consequences of insufficient water intake are truly devastating. It affects sight, muscle strength, kidney and liver function, heart beat rate, blood flow, and many others. We are constantly being reminded of the importance of clean, drinking water and yet people come to gyms for workout sessions or are running or cycling in nature without a bottle of water as if they came just to stand there and not to perform any kind of activity. The purpose of exercising is lost if the body ends up being dehydrated. Electrolyte-filled drinks and plain water are often what the body really needs to survive workout sessions.

Chapter 20: How Important Is Motivation For Your Workout?

So far, we have talked about several aspects of healthy living, as well as several aspects of exercising. However, one very important thing was not previously talked about in depth, and that is motivation. Every single one of us has been in a situation in which motivation for a workout was an issue, and all of us struggled to find motivation to return to training or take up some new activity. This section will try to explain what motivation is and how it can be reclaimed.

Sometimes, staying healthy or losing weight is not good enough motivation to get up early in the morning when it is raining outside and the temperature is freezing cold. In such cases, additional motivation is needed in order to follow you workout schedule and not fall behind in your exercise routines. It often happens that one skipped workout session can lead to a second, a second one leads to a third, and without you even realizing it, you have lost the habit of exercising and all the good things that came with it.

There are times when people will say things that will only make you doubt yourself. They might say things about you that you've been thinking for a long time. These types of things will make you lose all motivation to work out or do whatever it is that you are trying to do. You need to block those people out. If all they can say to you is about things you need to work on or things you aren't good enough at, you shouldn't be talking to them. Most of the time, their aim is to bring you down. They don't care if it what they say hurts you; they would rather make you feel bad about yourself. Sometimes, they are the ones doubting themselves. You should try your hardest to stick with your gut feeling, and don't give up. It will only lead to failure, and that's the last thing you want.

Another reason you might have a lack of motivation is if you have depression. Battling with depression is something so many people have to undergo on a daily basis. It is a lot of hard work, and sometimes, it's hard for them to get out of bed in the morning. If you have even an ounce of energy, you should put that towards something you want to be able to do, whether it's a hobby or a goal that you are trying to achieve. Every day will be a struggle, but it doesn't have to be the thing that holds you back from everything you can do in life. If you can find that ounce of energy, and you really want to get into shape, try putting this energy into working out. There are many workouts that have had positive effects on people who have depression. This isn't to say that working out will cure your depression, but there's a possibility that you will be able to deal with some of your symptoms more easily or simply feel relief from your symptoms. If there is something in your life that has that kind of effect on you, you should try your hardest to get out of bed to go do it.

The important thing to have in mind as regards motivation is that we must have a goal that makes us do more in order to achieve more. Doing one thing and not seeing any improvement or new results will cause the situation to quickly become tiresome, and people very often lose motivation to persevere. Continually reinventing goals is something that makes us motivated and provides us with reasons to do certain things, whether to read, study, work, or even exercise.

Reward Yourself

One of the best ways to keep yourself motivated to exercise or do some other type of work is to reward yourself after the completion of the activity. If you have problems with getting out of bed and going for a run, get out of bed and prepare a healthy fruit shake or some other type of delicious meal or drink, and condition yourself to run in order to enjoy the prepared meal or drink. Keep reinventing the rewards so that you will be able to keep it interesting without losing motivation. Go shopping, go to a movie, have a drink with friends, or take a nap, but only do so after you have finished with your exercise activities or any other activities. This positive conditioning enables you to create a positive habit of doing something, and in this way, the given activity will become a routine part of your day after some time. Soon, you will not need any motivation for this activity. The reason for this is that you are not doing daily activities in the same way, and your brain looks forward to new things.

Exercise With Friends

Another excellent way of staying motivated to do some exercise is to perform that exercise with a group of friends. Often, doing certain things with a group of friends makes it interesting and prevents us from feeling like the activity is the same old boring routine, which will eventually result in the lack of motivation for that activity. Friends are also great because they can get you out of bed and encourage you to exercise with them. While you do not necessarily want your friends to guilt you into going exercising with them, as this could create a negative attitude toward exercising, you will be more likely to show up to a previously arranged meeting to work out if you know that other people are depending on you to be there.

Surround yourself with ambitious people whose goal is to improve their lives in every aspect because soon, your will realize that you have also started to think similarly and to aim at an improved life. It is always important to have someone to remind you of what your goals are because sometimes, you get lost in the world, and you forget the reason why you do certain things. Exercising with friends who have a positive attitude towards exercising and towards life, in general, is one of the best ways to realize your full potential and to be happy with what you have accomplished up to that point and with what you want to accomplish in the future.

Step-By-Step Approach

For so many of us, it is sometimes hard to even get out of the bed. In those moments, going out and exercising seems like the last thing we want to do. The best solution is to start your day step by step. Do not set a goal of exercising as soon as you open your eyes. Instead, take one step at the time. Wake up, get out of bed, have a cup of coffee, have breakfast, put on your workout clothes and shoes, and only after you have fully enjoyed the morning should you go and do some exercise. A step-by-step routine helps you to overcome the lack of motivation; it gets your heart beat rate slightly elevated, and you will feel much better knowing what you have accomplished that morning.

The step-by-step approach also applies to your exercise routine overall. Do not expect that you will be able to launch yourself into complicated, challenging, or high-intensity workouts right away if you are just starting out. Focus on beginner exercises that are easy to learn and perform, and make sure that you are doing these exercises properly. As your fitness level improves, you will be able to take on new and more complex exercises and increase the challenges offered by your workout routine.

If you start out with unrealistic goals, then you will not achieve those goals, and you will be discouraged. Set realistic goals for yourself, such that each goal that you accomplish will encourage you to reach your next goal. In this way, you will continue to improve and advance your fitness level.

This step-by-step approach does not have to be limited only to exercise and workout regimens. It can be applied to all aspects of our lives. It does not matter if you need the motivation to exercise, to do your work, to study, or anything else. A step-by-step approach is something worth noting and remembering because you can only benefit from it.

Keep Your Workout Clothes In Sight

One of the most specific ways of maintaining and recapturing motivation to do some exercises or to go to the local gym is to keep your workout clothes in sight. In this way, you will constantly be reminded of exercising and its benefits. Keep your workout clothes or your running shoes somewhere in plain sight so that you get constantly reminded of the training. You can keep your clothes or your shoes next to your bed, in front of the bathroom door, or near the doors of your closet – it really does not matter. What matters is that your brain gets constant information about exercising, which will create a habit of exercising. Soon, you will be in a situation in which you will not need any motivation boosts in order to perform certain activities.

This technique also helps because if it is easier to get into your workout clothes and out to wherever you are exercising – whether it is the gym, running track, yoga studio, or your home workout station – then it is more likely that you would actually put on the clothes and go. Having everything immediately available takes away one obstacle on those days when your motivation may be low, and just one obstacle might be enough to prevent you from getting to your workout.

Motivational Quotes Work, Too

One of the biggest clichés as regards motivation or the lack of it is motivational quotes. However, for many people, motivational quotes do the job. Find people who inspire you, read and listen what they have written or said, and implement that in your daily routines, whether it has to do with exercise or something else. Find quotes on the Internet, write them down, and leave them next to your mirror so that you can see them every time you looked at yourself in the mirror. These motivational quotes will give you the positive energy boost that you require and will make you feel much better, especially if they are about the goals that you set for yourself. Do not run away from motivational reading material. Use it to make your own experience better and easier. Watch motivational videos because after watching or reading material like that, your brain will want to accomplish similar results, and it will encourage you to perform whatever activities you need to perform. Do not limit yourself to your own experience. Broaden your experience and world view by conducting research on other people's lives and experiences. See what they did that made them successful in life, and try to apply that in your own life.

Do What You Like

Another important thing is to do what you like and not what others expect you to do or what anybody else wants. In the end, nobody else matters but you. If you find yourself in a situation in which you do something that is not a pleasure for you, try to look around and see if what you have been doing is for you or for someone else. What you need to realize is that you are the master of your destiny. You decide on what you want to do. If you want to go swimming, do it because you like it, and you think that it is beneficial for you. Otherwise, you might get into a situation where your life feels miserable just because you do not want to say no to a friend when he or she invites you to a weightlifting workout when you actually hate weightlifting.

Do not be afraid of having your own opinion and saying "no" to things you do not like and that you think might harm you, your body, or your health. Life is short – too short to spend on doing things you do not like. When you do things you actually like to do, your need for motivation will be reduced to a minimum. This happens because your brain ties things you like with positive effects, and because of that, you will be willing to do such activities without any problems.

Part of doing what you like is adding variety to your workout. Even if you start out doing an exercise that you absolutely love, chances are pretty good that if you do that exercise repeatedly, you might eventually start to get tired of it. This will not exactly encourage you to keep going, especially if you are bored with what you are doing. Changing up the type of exercise that you are doing can keep you excited and interested in your workouts, which makes it much more likely that you will keep the exercise routine going.

If you feel like you are starting to get bored, you might want to consider trying out a new class at your gym, buying a workout video, looking up some new floor or weight exercises, or trying out a new type of exercise that you've never considered before.

Positive Thinking

Although this way of being motivated may be characterized as something for people from the hippie movement, the power of positive thinking has been proven to help, even in some cases of diseases. There are numerous cases in which terminally ill people managed to overcome their diseases when everything else failed because they refused to give up. They kept their heads up and kept being positive, and they were rewarded for not giving up. To keep a positive attitude towards people and life, in general, is to live a healthy and fulfilled life.

Positive thinking provides you with enough positive energy to fulfill your daily responsibilities without getting tired or exhausted. Negative thinking equals negative energy. When you are thinking positively, everyone around you feels that, and they feed off that positive energy, which makes their days and lives more positive. On the other hand, negative thoughts create negative energy, which makes everyone around you feel negative and bad. By staying positive, you do not only have a positive attitude towards life, but your body and brain also do not need any additional motivation for your daily activities.

Positive thinking may actually be one of the best ways to remain motivated for your daily activities, including exercising. With positive thinking, you might actually be unstoppable because it makes you believe that you can overcome any kind of obstacle that life throws at you. Positive thinking is not just an idea put forward by some hippies from the Beatles era. Positive thinking is much more than that. It is a life philosophy and a way of life.

Realistic Goals

One of the crucial things for you not to lose motivation and maintain it throughout the entire workout process is having realistic goals. Do not start exercising, or anything else in life for that matter, with big goals that are too high because that is a definite road to failure and feeling miserable. Instead, set your goal to be more realistic in nature. Create a list of short-term goals or those that are possible to achieve in a short period of time. Basically, what you need to do is to create a "to-do list." In this way, you will be able to cross out the goals that you have achieved so far. Achieving goals has a tremendous psychological influence over the human brain and the human body, such that it makes you immediately go for another goal on the list.

Instead of creating a goal of losing 60 pounds in 4 months or any other unrealistic time frame, create a goal of losing 5 to 10 pounds per month. In this way, you won't have to wait 6 months to cross out this goal. Instead, you will be able to cross out one goal every month, and we already mentioned the psychological effects of achieving short-term goals. If you keep doing this, you will always have the motivation to perform certain activities, and it will provide you with the boost of positive energy that can only help you in further fulfilling of your goals. However, in a situation in which you wait for a long time in order to achieve your goal, your motivation decreases as time passes by. This is because if it takes you too long to achieve a goal, then the improvement is hardly visible, and you lose motivation when wondering what the point of all this is.

Lower Your Expectations

Strongly correlated with setting realistic goals is lowering your expectations as regards certain activities that you perform in your life. By lowering your expectations, you are taking the pressure off, which makes you perform your activities much more effectively and productively. When your expectations are too high and you fail to meet such expectations, your level of motivation will be very low, and it will become a problem for you to start doing something else.

On the other hand, every fulfilled expectation gives you a motivational boost that keeps you on the right track. Fulfilling your expectations also gives a boost of positive energy, which makes everything else feel better. No matter how small expectations are, the psychological effects of fulfilling such expectations do wonders relative to staying motivated for any other kind of activity in the future.

As mentioned previously, the issue of motivation can be crucially important in achieving goals and fulfilling your plans. However, there are often situations in which motivation is lacking, and we need to find a way to raise that level of motivation in order to fulfill and achieve previously determined plans. Several solutions to this kind of problem were given in this section. However, that does not mean that these solutions can be applied to your case because every person is different, and different things and customs make people motivated.

The aforementioned list is just an example of what some people have done to overcome their problems that were caused by the lack of motivation. The most important thing in all of this is that you do what you like and what makes you feel happy. This is the best possible way to stay motivated and avoid the problems caused by the lack of motivation.

Chapter 21: Stay In Shape Even When You Are On A Vacation

Everybody needs a vacation at least once a year. In those 10 to 15 days, the body and mind go through completely different processes than the ones they were used to before you go on a vacation. For people who are used to regular exercising, going on a vacation can be slightly problematic because their daily routine will be interrupted, and that can sometimes prove to be bad for the body. If you spend a lot of time working out and exercising, your body has already gotten used to the physical effort that has been put into the workout. However, a sudden change of routine – from daily workouts to 10 to 15 days of no workout – can be slightly problematic for the body. There is no evidence of the medical consequence of pausing workout sessions. However, psychologically, it might feel at least a bit unusual to spend 10 to 15 days without any workout being done. With the lack of adequate equipment, the lack of time, or any other reason, working out when on a vacation has proven to be a challenge not everyone is equipped to face.

In order to stay in shape when you almost have no means of doing that, you must look for alternative ways of exercising. Your standard workout might seem difficult after returning from vacation, but do not worry because while you were on vacation, your body got used to slightly fewer sessions, but you will be in the same old form after only a couple of days. Make sure that you find an exercise that suits you and the needs of your body because sometimes, mistakes can lead to injuries and a total pause from workout regimes. All the things you did for preparation before the workout must be done again when you are on a vacation because doing any type of exercise without proper pre-warm up exercises is risky, and you can end up suffering from injuries that can cause a lot of problems and keep you out of the gym for a longer period of time.

Eat Enough Protein

One of the ways in which you can maintain the strength of your body while on vacation is to eat a lot of proteins. Food that contains a lot of protein can be found in every store, so you do not have to worry about whether you will be able to find any protein-rich food. When talking about protein-rich food, it is important to emphasize that the greatest amount of protein can be found in meat, cheese, fish, different kinds of seeds, nuts, and eggs. That being said, it is important to emphasize that you must be careful with this kind of food because too much of anything can have completely different results than what is desired. It is also very important to stay properly hydrated or to drink enough water, because the lack of water in human body takes its toll on muscle strength. When there isn't enough water in the human body, muscles lose their strength, and the body becomes tired very quickly. Having a hydrated body might also give you some motivation to go to the gym. You'll feel good, but you know that you'll feel even better once you've completed a workout.

Improvise

When all fails, your improvisation and imagination might help you in a way you would never expect. When faced with the lack of opportunity to work out, similar effects can be simulated by doing some other activities. For example, start walking more. Go out for longer walks. In doing so, your body will work out just enough to maintain the level of readiness you had before going on a vacation. Heavy traveling bags can sometimes be used to train your biceps and triceps for them to remain lean and strong. If it happens that you are vacationing near a mountain, go for a hike. The effort you put into hiking will get your heart beat rate up, increase blood flow, and enable you to sustain the level of physical readiness you had before going on a vacation. If it happens that you are vacationing somewhere on the seashore, swimming is the best option for you and your muscles. Another great vacation exercise is playing different sports. There is likely to be a sports court within the vicinity. Whether it is basketball, football, soccer, beach volleyball, tennis court, or something else, sports are a great way of staying in shape and maintaining muscle integrity.

Find A Local Gym

A local gym is always a great idea for continuing your workout sessions. In this case, there is no need to change any aspect of the workout just because you are traveling. One of the problems with finding a local gym in the place where you are staying is the fact that you will have to pay a membership fee in order for you to use its services. Everything that you did in the gym in your hometown, you can also do in the gym where you are on vacation. Ask around, and see whether the hotel you are staying in has a gym or pool. Swimming would be an excellent activity for preserving the strength of your muscles while providing you with the opportunity to work on your cardio. Finding a local gym would be an ideal replacement when you go on a vacation. However, that is sometimes impossible, so you would be forced to find another way to work on your physical readiness.

In recent years, another type of workout has become more and more popular, and that is the street workout. Using bars and other elements placed publicly on the streets, it is possible to maintain your form, as well as build stronger and leaner muscles from scratch. The street workout is an efficient way of working out, but it is also very demanding, and it requires adequate preparation just like the case with all other exercises.

Fitness Classes

If you are staying at a resort, or even if you are on a cruise ship, there are often fitness classes that are offered to guests. In addition to being a great option for getting in some exercise, it is also a good way to meet fellow guests and some locals and to make friends during your vacation. Moreover, you might be exposed to the local culture if it is incorporated into the fitness classes. For example, in Cuba, many resorts offer classes that introduce traditional Cuban dances, such as salsa and rumba, as part of workout routines. There are almost always fitness classes available, no matter where you are. These can open your eyes to a whole new realm of exercises that you can try out. Some of them might feel strange, but there will be some that will connect with you, and you might bring that into your workout, enhancing it with something fun and exciting. This can help bring your workout routine from just a routine to something that will make you smile.

Work Out In Your Hotel Room

Your hotel room is also a very good place where you can do a certain number of exercises that will enable you to maintain your fitness and workout sessions. Several pieces of equipment used for exercising are portable, so you can bring them with you on your travels. One such piece of equipment is a jump rope, the role and importance of which have been mentioned previously. Notably, 30 minutes of exercising with a jump rope is sometimes more useful than an hour of running, swimming, or cycling. Aside from jumping rope, you can do a lot more exercises that will make your muscles strong and lean, as well as preserve the level of their strength until you can return to your previously determined workout regimen. Some of these exercises include squats, burpees, pushups, crunches, and many others.

Moreover, if you have enough space in your traveling bags, you could carry a bar for chin-ups. Sometimes, chin-ups can be done by only using a door frame. As discussed earlier in the book, resistance bands are a great option for exercising while traveling because they are very light and take up virtually no room in your luggage. These exercises will not only preserve the strength of your muscles but will also improve your heart beat rate and blood flow, as well as increase the intake of oxygen necessary for the proper functioning of the human body.

Jumping jacks are also a very good choice, not only for working out when you are on vacation, but also when you are not because your whole body gains benefits while doing jumping jacks, as almost every muscle is involved in the performance of this exercise.

Aside from the already mentioned exercises, push-ups are also among the most effective one, yet they are very simple, and because of that, they can be performed almost under all circumstances and in all locations. This makes them a great exercise to perform while on vacation. Moreover, many hotels have a fitness room, so you should definitely utilize that. They generally come with a treadmill, maybe an elliptical, a bike, and maybe some free weights, but this is more than enough to do a simple workout.

There are also hotels that have pools. If the pool is indoors, you don't have to worry about the time of year. Swimming is a wonderful exercise, and if you have access to a pool or any body of water to swim in, you should definitely try to take advantage of that. You'll feel better about not being able to perform your typical routine if you get a good workout doing something.

While you are on vacation, the intensity and duration of your workout are significantly reduced because you are limited in term of the resources that are available to you at that time. Depending on whom you are with while vacation, it is always better to spend more time with friends or family than doing too much exercise that is not adjusted to your needs. If you decide that you would continue with the workout while on vacation, you need to make a commitment because it is very easy to find excuses for not working out, and this is especially easy when you are visiting new cities or new countries.

There is one problem with working out while you are on vacation. Give that you are on vacation, you should be relaxing and enjoying some free time. Otherwise, the purpose of the entire vacation seems pointless. You should work out, but you should also have a lot of time to relax and enjoy the scenery, food, company, and everything that comes with vacation because without a healthy mind, the health of the body has no purpose. If your vacation is somewhere that you'll be spending a lot of time on a beach or somewhere that you'll be swimming, you should take full advantage of that. Swimming is a workout, yes, but you'll have fun doing it. If you're with your family, then going to a beach or a pool is even more beneficial. Everyone can have a fun time, and you can still get your workout in without leaving them.

Although the medical aspects of interrupting continuous workout sessions reveal no serious problems, it may be hard for you to find motivation to get back to training after you have returned from a vacation where you have not spent any time exercising. Given that the lack of motivation can be crucial in maintaining a healthy lifestyle, it is important to have at least the smallest habit of waking up early, eating healthy food, doing some cardio, and preserving the strength and integrity of your muscles.

While it can be difficult to resist overeating or eating unhealthy foods while you are on vacation, you should try and avoid doing so for the most part. It is okay to indulge every once in a while, but if you indulge in every meal the whole time that you are traveling, it is going to have a significant negative impact on your diet and can set you back quite a bit. Focus on eating vegetables, fruits, and baked or grilled foods, and remember that you do not need to eat dessert after every meal. Healthy options are almost always available. You just have to pay attention to your options, and pick the foods that will fit in best with your dietary plan.

A vacation is a time to enjoy and relax, but that does not mean that you have to give up your fitness goals completely while you are away. You will feel better about yourself and enjoy your time more if you try and stick with your regimen as much as you can while still taking advantage of the opportunities that present themselves during your vacation.

Key Highlights

Weight loss is a very important aspect of life. If you are fat or obese, then it is high time that you decide to put your health back on the right track. The best way to know whether you are overweight is by checking your body mass index. You should be within your minimum limits. You need to check your weight and then calculate your BMI. Even if you are in the right range, it is important to take care of your body. It does not take a lot to tone your body; all you need is a little dedication. Once you get the hang of it, you will continue to pursue it and get your body into good shape. Your confidence level will increase, and you will have a chance to live a better life.

Nutrition is key when you wish to lose weight or maintain a slim figure. You must look at what you are putting into your body. You cannot blindly follow a diet just because someone else is seeing positive results with it. You must come up with a meal plan that is beneficial to you. As mentioned in this book, you need to calculate the calories needed by your body and consume no more than necessary. You must also take care of the fat that you are consuming, and try to limit the bad fat while promoting the good fat. Try and eat as much healthy and nutritious food as possible, and don't include any junk food. If you are finding it tough to stay away from junk food, then consider having just one cheat meal per week.

Being vegan or vegetarian doesn't mean that you can't be just as lean and fit as everyone else. In fact, many people have switched to this kind of lifestyle and have had some really amazing results. Many times, it changed their life so much that they start losing weight because they cleansed their body of a lot of the processed foods they had been eating. Being a vegan or vegetarian is a huge change in your life, but you can still work out and lose weight. You can feel really good about yourself and know that your reasons for going down this route are your own. No one will be able to change that fact.

Exercise is a must, no matter how fit you already are. By exercising, you will do your body a whole host of good. You will have the chance to have better heart health, increase your immunity, and remain active for longer periods of time. You can choose any cardio exercise, like running or swimming, if you do not have the time to perform the prescribed exercises in this book. If you do decide on this, remember that there is no point in not taking them up. It's now or never, so it is best that you start exercising at the earliest possible time, and reap its benefits.

Supplements are necessary to consume as your body might not get the needed nutrition solely through the food you consume. You need to supplement your food with supplements loaded with nutrients and multivitamins. You can choose any of the nutrients mentioned in this book to help boost your weight loss and muscle gain. However, you might have to consult a physician first in order to remain safe from any side effects. Overdosing will not help you see faster results, so it is important to remain within the prescribed limits.

The recipes mentioned in this book will be great to start with, but you must not limit yourself to just those on the list. You must come up with recipes that suit your taste and palate. The ultimate goal is to remain healthy for life, so you need to make the consumption of healthy foods a lifestyle choice. If you are having difficulty understanding what needs to be added to your meals to benefit your weight loss regimen, then you can work with a nutritionist and come up with a list of foods that are good for you.

Meal frequency needs to be worked on if you wish to reduce your weight and increase your metabolism. You really should get over the "eat three meals a day" to remain healthy theory, and take up the five to six meal plan. You can split your three meals into five to six meals, and make sure you are not overeating. Again, you can work closely with a nutritionist and come up with a meal plan that works best for your body.

Stopping with bad habits, such as smoking and drinking, will go a long way in helping you remain fit and healthy for life.

Alternative exercises, such as Pilates and yoga, are a must for all-around body development. Sticking to hardcore exercises alone will not do your body any good. You need to focus on mixing it up with relaxing exercise routines that will work on your brain and body. Try and do yoga at least five times a week. You can choose alternate days. You can also introduce breathing exercises that will help you feel relaxed and remain motivated.

It is extremely important to have all your vital statistics checked and recorded before you choose to take up weight loss as a mission. You should have your weight, blood pressure, glucose levels, and other such important statistics measured and recorded. You must tell your physician that you are taking up a diet and an exercise routine to lose weight. Once you get the go signal, you can start practicing the exercises and reel in good health. Remember to monitor your stats from time to time, and it is best that you buy yourself a weight machine, a blood pressure monitoring machine, and a blood sugar monitor to remain healthy.

Remember to never give up on anything that you take up. It is a tough task to lose weight and remain fit, no doubt, but you must persevere and not give up just because you seek faster results. If you put in the hard work, then you will definitely see good results. It's just a matter of time, and once you see results, you will continue to work hard. If you are having problems continuing, then convince someone to take up the diet and exercise program with you. The two of you will motivate each other to continue doing the good work. You can also join a group session, like a yoga class, or simply join a gym to motivate you.

Rewarding yourself from time to time is vital. You need to give yourself a gift in order to remain motivated. You can gift yourself something material or simply hit the spa. As long as you look forward to getting the gift, you will be motivated to put in the hard work. However, you must remember not to do it often, as it might end up becoming a common thing. So set yourself yearly or half-yearly goals in terms of your weight loss, and once you successfully achieve these goals, buy yourself something valuable.

Conclusion

Thank you again for purchasing this book!

I really hope this book was able to help you understand how fitness nutrition works so that you can achieve your weight loss and fitness goals. I have tried my best to motivate you into taking up nutrition to attain a healthy body.

The next step is to start making improvements in your diet and daily routine by putting all that you have learned from this book into action. There is no better time than now to get started on a healthier and more active lifestyle.

If you've enjoyed this book, then I'd like to ask you for a favor. Would you be kind enough to leave a review for this book on Amazon? It'd be greatly appreciated!

Thank you, and good luck!

Nicholas Bjorn

FREE E-BOOKS SENT WEEKLY

Join <u>North Star Readers Book Club</u>
And Get Exclusive Access To The Latest Kindle Books in
Fitness, Health, Weight Loss and Much More...

TO GET YOU STARTED HERE IS YOUR FREE E-BOOK:

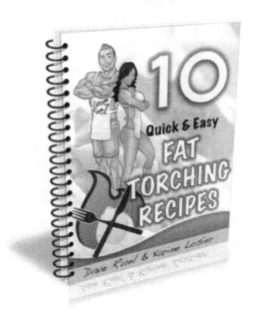

Visit to Sign Up Today!

www.northstarreaders.com/10-fat-torching-recipes

HAVE YOU BEEN DREAMING SO LONG ABOUT HAVING TONED AND WELL-DEFINED MUSCLES?

DO YOU HAVE NO IDEA OF HOW YOU CAN START ACHIEVING THE BODY OF YOUR DREAMS?

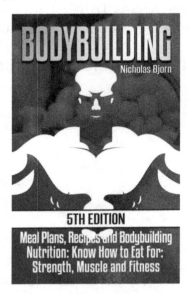

The good news is that this book can show you how! Bulking up and maintaining a toned physique cannot be easily accomplished without the right plan and discipline. Most of all, a definitive guide can go a long way in walking you through the steps you need to take to achieve your bodybuilding goals.

Here's what this book will teach you:
- What bodybuilding is
- Why bodybuilding is good for you
- How you should set your bodybuilding goals
- What nutrients you need for bodybuilding
- What characteristics your meal plan should have
- How to draw up a nutritional bodybuilding plan

Bodybuilding and meal planning are made a breeze through the tips and sample plans presented in this book!

Visit to Order Your Copy Today!
www.amazon.com/dp/1515364003

SO YOU'VE BEEN EATING HEALTHY AND WORKING OUT TO ACHIEVE YOUR FITNESS GOALS, BUT DO YOU FEEL AS IF YOU NEED A GREATER BOOST IN YOUR NUTRITION?

DO YOU THINK THAT WHAT YOU'RE DOING AND WHAT YOU'RE CONSUMING ARE JUST NOT ENOUGH?

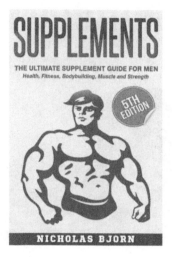

Most men dream of having a sculpted physique that simply screams "Alpha Male." But sometimes, gaining lean muscle is not as simple as a healthy diet and a regular workout regimen. The good news is that you can get that boost you need through supplementation, and this book can show you how!

Here is what this book will help you learn:
- Ranking the top 10 supplements for men
- The benefits of each of these supplements
- Proper dosage to get the optimum results
- Safety precautions to avoid any side effects

Take the necessary steps to achieve the sculpted physique that you've always wanted to achieve.

Visit to Order Your Copy Today!
www.amazon.com/dp/1530753945

GOOD NUTRITION IS IMPORTANT – THIS IS A FACT.

BUT HOW DO YOU REALLY GET STARTED TO ACHIEVING IT? PEOPLE SAY IT BEGINS WITH A BALANCED DIET, BUT HOW EXACTLY DO YOU ACHIEVE THAT BALANCE?

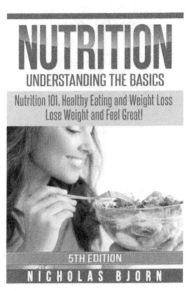

If you are lost in the world of calories and kilojoules, this book is the perfect reference to help you! The contents of this book will help you focus on what's important while getting rid of all the unnecessary fluff about dieting and healthy living that are just bound to confuse you.

Here is what this book has in store for you:
- Nutrition defined and simplified
- Dietary guidelines made easy to follow
- Nutrition labels made understandable
- Vitamins and minerals explained
- Fat-burning foods enumerated
- Meal planning and recipes made doable

Start reaping the benefits of eating healthy and living healthy! You can get started today.

Visit to Order Your Copy Today!
www.amazon.com/dp/1519485492

Made in United States
Orlando, FL
14 January 2024